NO MORE FEAR

Sexual Assault and the Four "C's" of Rape Avoidance

Second Edition

Stephen M. Thompson

KENDALL/HUNT PUBLISHING COMPANY
4050 Westmark Drive Dubuque, Iowa 52002

To
"Chubby" and "Bud"

ISBN 0-8403-8201-4

Printed in the United States of America
10 9 8 7 6 5 4 3

CONTENTS

PREFACE

Rape—perhaps one of the strongest, most emotion provoking words in our language today. Only a short time ago, few of us were touched by the trauma of rape. Today, however, most of us know someone who has been a victim. She is no longer a faceless object; she is a wife, daughter, mother, or friend.

The odds are that more than one out of two women will experience a sexual assault situation sometime in her life. Of those, half will avoid the rapist and the other half will not.

The problem today is that there are so many strategies being taught to women to avoid rape, that it is confusing. How does one choose? Who or what does one believe?

Throughout this book, I will present to you a realistic, highly successful system of avoiding rape. I will not be telling you to scream, kick the knee, punch the nose, throw up on the man, or any number of other relatively unsuccessful techniques that other ''experts'' are advising you to do. You will be given a system of avoidance that will make sense, be easy to use, increase your confidence, and most importantly, give you the option to win.

In the following chapters, you will learn a system of rape avoidance that is being used today by thousands of females. It has taken years of research including over 5,000 interviews with victims and rapists, experimental studies, and countless hours of thought and frustration in order to develop this system.

The Four ''C's'' are designed to counter the actions of a rapist. Briefly, your first 'C'—Concern for Personal Safety is designed so that you greatly minimize the chance of ever being selected by a rapist as a victim. If, however, you are selected, your second and third ''C's''—Confidence and Control are designed to eliminate most potentially aggressive situations. Rapists expect the woman to either fight or be frightened. In this option, you take control of him and the situation without having to rely on physical techniques. If the situation is such that confidence and control are not effective, or you are not given a chance to use them, Complete Incapacitation can then be used. There are only two techniques taught in this 'C'. They are simple, avoid confusion, and are 100 percent incapacitating if you use them.

I believe it is important to note that the term avoidance is used frequently throughout the book. Avoidance is what intended victims do to stop the assault. Prevention is what needs to be done to get at the cause of violence towards women. Prevention stops the assailant from starting his assaultive behavior. Women avoid rape—only men can prevent it!

This book was created to give you knowledge and confidence without producing fear. You will learn what some of the motivating factors are that cause men to rape; you will see that, in reality, there are two distinctly different types of rapes; you will understand the method by which rapists select a woman and ultimately sexually assault her; and you will learn what *really* works to defeat them and what does not! Finally, you will be able to eliminate your fears of sexual assault, for you will have the best weapon available with which to win—yourself.

ACKNOWLEDGMENTS

I want to thank everyone who has helped me make this book a reality, especially: Meg Rouleau; Carole Howard; Raymond Sinclair; and my wife, Linda. Photography by Robert Barclay. Cover idea by Dennis Focken.

CHAPTER

1

THE TYPES OF STRANGER RAPISTS AND THE RAPE SEQUENCE

The threat of sexual assault (rape) hangs over every female in our society regardless of age, career, style of dress, or socioeconomic level. This threat is based upon the plain fact that approximately one in two women in our society will some day encounter a sexual assault situation. They do not make glaring headlines, but they do scar our society and the people who live in it.

Prior to the mid-1970's, few of us actually knew a victim of rape. She was a headline, undoubtedly someone who was asking for it, a tramp—never us. However, today, we are much closer to the problem because we probably know a victim. Perhaps she is a sister, daughter, mother, or friend. We see that she is just like us and we are forced to admit that we could also become victims. We prefer to think that bad things always happen to someone else. Unfortunately, we are all somebody else's someone else.

As the visibility and awareness of sexual assault increases, so does the need to understand the crime and combat it. The first step in understanding the crime is to identify the various types of rapists. Many people, unfortunately, place rapists into one generic group believing that they are all alike and are motivated by the same needs. For example, a female is outside her apartment and a male approaches her; they talk for a minute or two and then he grabs at her breasts; she yells at him while slapping his face and he turns and runs. This would be classified as a sexual assault and the male labeled as a rapist. Two nights later, a woman is approached the same way, but this victim is beaten, thrown to the ground and forcibly penetrated. That too, is classified as a sexual assault and the male labeled a rapist. Are they the same? NO!! In reality, these are two completely different types of sexual assaults— different intensities of motives, attitudes, and different personalities involved. Once able to understand this, you will be better prepared to analyze the proper course of action to defeat the assailant. What works against one type of rapist may not work against another.

TYPE I—SEXUAL CONFRONTATION

The *Sexual Confronter* is a male motivated by the need to control and sexually dominate a female. He sees her as an object, something to be used and then discarded. He may meet a female and within a short time attempt to sexually violate her through initiating some form of intimidation. If she responds negatively in the form of a scream, a slap or kick, or an assertive no, he will most often stop and seek out a different victim. If, however, she is intimidated by his actions, he will continue. It is imperative that you remember, most sexual confronters are not out to fight. He will usually not resort to violence to get what he wants. He is motivated by the need to assume power and control over a female through sexual domination.

Violence, for the sake of clarification, is defined as the intent to do bodily harm to the female in the form of hitting, stabbing, etc. While aggression is present in all assaults, not all rapists are motivated by the need to inflict physical pain.

TYPE II—VIOLENT SEXUAL ATTACK

The *Violent Sexual Attacker* is a male motivated by the need to have power and control over a female, while at the same time directing violence and sexual degradation toward her. His goal is to dominate, humiliate, and show the female that he is the one who controls. He does not generally kill, because he wants the female to live with the fact that she was beaten and defiled.

Strong evidence is pointing to the fact that there are really two, Type II personalities. As was just described, the first one vents his hatred through violence directed at the female, without intending to kill her. The second Type II personality has the desire to murder as an additional motive.

So, as you see, we are dealing, on the street, with rapists driven by different motives. While Type I's motives are power, control, and sexual domination; the Type II is motivated not only by these, but also by violence.

When describing strategies of rape avoidance, women are usually taught to use techniques to defend against the crime of sexual assault, unaware of the fact that they are dealing with essentially, two different types of rapists. Where a slap, scream, or other assertive, confrontational behavior will most often defeat a Type I, the same action directed against either of the Type II personalities, may well elicit a drastically different response; a response based on hatred, violence, the drive to dominate, degrade, and possibly, murder. This type of rapist cannot allow himself to be defeated by the female.

RAPE SEQUENCE

Now that you have a basic understanding that there are different motives for rape, let's now look at the process of rape—that is, what steps does a rapist go through to create a victim. Over the past 15 years, I have interviewed thousands of victims and rapists. A pattern of rape behavior was apparent, but it was not until Dr. James Selkins' ''Behavioral Analysis of Rape,'' that this pattern was identified in terms of a specific sequence that rapists follow. By knowing the rape sequence, you will be able to understand how the rapist works, and what is necessary to avoid becoming a victim.

The Rape Sequence is made up of five stages; stages which are based on a behavioral progression. The first stage, is called *Target Selection*. Before a rape can take place, the male must first choose a victim. How does he choose? The key word used when selecting his victim is VULNERABILITY. Vulnerability can pertain to the victim's environment, her age, personality, or any number of other factors that would meet the rapist's definition of a vulnerable female. It is vulnerability that determines why one woman is raped and another not! As examples, a female alone is much more vulnerable than one in the company of others. A female who walks with her head down, submissively, is more likely to be selected than a woman who walks briskly and with confidence, and so on.

Once the rapist has selected a possible victim, he then moves into the next stage of the sequence—*Approach/Test*.

There are two factors involved with the *Approach/Test*. In the first, the rapist is attempting to get close to his victim without alarming her. His goal is to get less than an arms distance away from her. In the second, as he is approaching her, he is talking with her—testing to see if he can dominate and control her. Perhaps his victim is in a store parking lot, with no one around. He walks up to her, all the while disarming her through asking questions about the store, etc. Does she stop and answer his questions while allowing him to get close? If so, she is being successfully *Approach/Tested*.

Testing takes many forms depending upon the particular situation. One victim I interviewed related that she was in a lounge, with some friends, when a male asked her to dance. After they danced, she allowed the man to lead her over to his table and buy her a drink. He asked her name, where she lived, if she lived alone, etc. She refused his offer of a second drink, however, he purchased it anyway saying that she didn't want to hurt his feelings, and she drank it (test). A short while later, her friends told her they were going to leave. The man stated that he would like to take her out for some coffee, and that he would see that she got home (test). She accepted his offer and they left. Instead of going in the direction of a restaurant, the male went in a different direction. The female asked where he was going and he stated that he had coffee in his apartment (test). He than said, "What's the matter, don't you trust me?" Though uncomfortable, she went along with him. Once in the apartment, he progressed rapidly through the other steps in the sequence, and she was brutalized and became a victim of rape.

Another victim interviewed, allowed a man into her apartment who told her he was taking a survey. She let him in instead of talking outside or saying no. She answered a few questions, got him a soft drink, and ultimately became a victim.

Remember that there are many ways of testing, but the main factor is the male's ability to elicit submissive behavior from the female while getting close to her. He knows that first, most people don't believe they will ever be victims of anything; and secondly, most people are uncomfortable when they feel they have made someone else uncomfortable. Consequently, victims tend to become vulnerable because they want to avoid the discomfort created by letting the man know he is not trusted. It is also extremely important to realize that most rapes begin with talking. The male is close to you and you have little idea that he is a rapist until. . . .

After the female has passed his test, and he is close to her the male progresses to the next step in the sequence—*Intimidation.* If a woman can be intimidated, the rape will proceed to its final conclusion. Intimidation brings forth the display of illegal behavior on the part of the male. The rapist may grab, hit, threaten, use vulgar language, and/or anything else he sees as intimidating. Most Sexual Confronters will not use violence to intimidate. They may threaten certain things, but will not follow through with the threats if the woman resists. A few of these rapists may use violence as a means of retaliating—she fights, he fights back until she is intimidated, and then he stops. The Violent Sexual Attacker however, will use violence because it is one of his primary motives.

In the intimidation stage, the male will make his demands known to the female. He indicates at this point, what the punishment will be if she refuses to cooperate, and what her reward will be if she does cooperate. Remember, most Type I's will leave if they see that the female cannot be intimidated into fulfilling their needs. The Violent Sexual Attacker (Type II) will not give up attempting to intimidate the female until they have succeeded, or until they have been completely incapacitated by her.

Once the victim has been intimidated, the *Sexual Violation* occurs. It is the rapist's behavior during this stage that reveals the inner being—his needs, fears, and fantasies. Victims have described a great variety of behaviors from boasting (demanding the victim respond as if she is pleased), to extreme violence. There are no boundaries to the behavior of the rapist nor to his demands during this stage of the sequence.

The final stage in the sequence of rape is *Termination.* This is generally accomplished in one of three ways. The male may continue his intimidation by threatening to come back and harm her or her family, if she goes to the police. It must be pointed out that this is the most common method of terminating by strangers, and for the most part, it is a bluff. I have found that there is a greater chance the male will come back if you do not go to the police than if you do. The reason is simple—he does not have to test or intimidate because he has already accomplished them. When he returns he will begin with *Sexual Violation.* An assault victim I talked with in California, was sexually assaulted several times by the same man. Every time he terminated he said he would kill her children if she went to the police. She finally couldn't cope any longer and reported the assaults. They caught the rapist and convicted him.

A second method of terminating used is to appeal to the female's sympathy by crying, apologizing, pleading for understanding, or by playing on her guilt by trying to make her feel responsible for his actions. This method is used quite often, especially if she knows the male.

The final method of termination is accomplished by attempting to kill the victim. Though not always successful in murdering the victim, the rapist feels that if the woman is dead she cannot be a witness. Whatever the method of termination, the goal is to prevent the woman from reporting the assault.

SUMMARY

Remember, rapists follow a pattern of behavior which is called the Rape Sequence. Though we do not know specifically *what* a rapist will do, we have a good idea *how* he thinks and acts. For any rape avoidance strategy to be effective, you must break out of this sequence—no matter whether you're dealing with a Type I (non-violent) or Type II (violent) rapist!!

The Four 'C's' is the only rape avoidance strategy designed to break the rape sequence before you become a victim. Read on and learn!!

Chapter 1 Worksheet

What is the major difference between Sexual Confronters, and Violent Sexual Attackers?

What is the rapist looking for in Target Selection?

Explain Approach/Test.

Give an example of how a rapist would go through the first three steps of the sequence using a location or scenario that you know.

CHAPTER

2

FAMILIAR (DATE/ACQUAINTANCE) RAPE: The Most Prevalent Type I Rapist

There is much being said today about date/acquaintance rape. The reality is that approximately 60% of all rapists are known to their victims. He may be a date, friend of a friend, co-worker, or simply the nice man who works or lives next door. Who is this man, this predator?

In talking with victims about the familiar rapist, they consistently refer to him as such a nice guy. The type of person no one would guess could resort to such abhorrent behavior. It is just this misconception that causes people to blame the victim and somehow justify holding her responsible for his behavior. "She shouldn't have dressed that way!" "What could she expect, having a drink and going back to his place. She asked for it." With victim blaming statements such as these, is it any wonder why so few women report this crime!

Let's look at who this "nice guy" is and how he assaults. The more you know about this man, the easier it will be to avoid him.

"NICE GUY" PROFILE

Though every rapist is unique in his own right, there are several characteristics that are common among familiar rapists.

He will generally display some or all of the following traits:

- Macho, athletic and outwardly confident. Probably was a high school athlete.

- Attractive and well liked by females. He has no trouble getting close to women.

- He tends to need to be around men in groups. It is likely that he would be in a fraternity, civic organization, athletic team, or sport club. He is the kind of man who would organize a softball team for a summer league. He makes frequent stops to the bar to be around friends.

- He is, most likely, not married. He is not inclined to enter into long term relationships.

As you can see, this male seems like the all-American kind of guy. Everybody likes him—few would believe he is capable of rape! However, underneath this likeable exterior, there are other traits that are not so obvious. These following traits are the ones that will determine that this "nice guy" will become something more—a rapist.

- Egocentric, self-serving, and feels little guilt.

- Brags about his female conquests.

- He has a very difficult time with criticism or rejection. This may explain why he tries so hard to be liked.
- He will almost always "score" or rape by the third time he is with the woman in an environment where there is little or no chance anyone will hear.
- He believes he has the right to be aggressive to get what he wants.
- He tends to be socially immature.
- This man is aroused by portrayals in which a rape victim consistently abhorred the experience.

RAPE SEQUENCE OF THE FAMILIAR RAPIST

Now that you have an idea of who this person is, let us examine how he accomplishes the assault.

He will generally select someone that is in his own age range and socio-economic bracket. A college student is likely to target a college student. A professional on Wall Street would be most inclined to select a woman that works on Wall Street, etc. His selection is made through incidental contact. She is a friend of a friend, or possibly someone he has seen before through work or during leisure hours. He will attempt to strike up a conversation with her. There is something about her that attracts him. He senses that he will be able to get her to trust him. Frequently he is attracted to the female who appears to have consumed the most alcohol—he thinks this makes her more easily led (vulnerable).

Once he has selected a potential conquest (victim), he attempts to get her attracted to him. He will be very nice and attentive, yet always attempting to control her and the situation. He frequently uses alcohol as a means to test her control and to make her more submissive. She feels no threat because of who he is, and the fact that people are around.

While he is testing her he will be desensitizing her to him. He will do such things as joke with her while touching her arm. In other words, he is trying to intrude on her space without alarming her. If successful, he will escalate. His behavior may become slightly inappropriate. A hand lingering on her arm or leg. Maybe his language changes and he swears or tells an "off-color" joke. His hand may "accidentally" brush her breast, or touch her somewhat inappropriately while dancing. He makes calculated moves to determine if she is ready.

Once he determines that the time is right, he will suggest they go somewhere more private to talk, listen to music, have a drink, or a variety of other ploys designed to separate her from people who could give support. Most often this location is his residence.

Once this "nice guy" gets the woman to an isolated environment, he will become sexually aggressive. His goal is a sexual conquest! If the woman *willingly* complies, he sees it as a "score." If, however, she resists, he will negotiate. If that does not work he will try to pressure her. If that fails he will become very aggressive and use whatever means necessary to intimidate her so that he can take what he wants.

In this phase of intimidation, there are no rules. He will increase his force based on the resistance given by the victim. Though he does not initiate violent behavior, he will retaliate with it to get what he wants.

After he has intimidated her, he will enter into the sexual violation phase of the rape. He will generally be aggressive and demanding. He will take what he wants with little regard for her.

The final phase of his rape sequence involves Termination. If the female has willingly complied, he will continue with the nice guy behavior by taking her home, etc. He will usually leave her with the idea that he will call her. It is unlikely that he will see her again. However, if he had to intimidate her to accomplish his conquest, his termination will be to threaten the victim and/or, blame her for what has occurred.

His threats can be physical, but generally his termination technique is to convince her that no one will believe her. He says he will tell people she wanted it—she had drinks with him, went back to his place, and had sex with him. He may also use blame and guilt with statements like, "Why did you let me buy you those drinks and then come home with me? You teased me! You wanted it and you know it!'' He will attempt to convince her that she brought this on herself.

The familiar rapist is motivated by the conquest through sexual domination. If she is a willing participant, great. If she resists, well that is okay too! He feels entitled and that what he has done is not wrong—not rape. The goal to him is the conquest!

SUMMARY

Familiar rape is a crime of tremendous proportions. It is unlikely that there is any crime more under-reported than this, nor victims more persecuted than these. The ``nice guy'' finds a victim, gets close to her through being attentive and nice, gets her alone, and then does whatever is necessary to put another notch on the bed post. He then goes on his way to prey upon someone else, leaving this woman victimized and struggling to cope with something few of us understand.

Chapter 2 Worksheet

List as many characteristics to the profile of the Familiar rapist as you can remember.

Why do you think he is so successful as a rapist?

How does his Rape Sequence differ from the Stranger rapist?

CHAPTER

3

RAPE AVOIDANCE STRATEGIES

I really sympathize with a woman who is attempting to become more educated about rape avoidance. There is a lot of advice being given so, who do you listen to, who do you believe? Let's examine rape avoidance, the evolution of it and where we are today.

It is very important to understand that *all* methods have their successes and proponents. What we must look at is SUCCESS RATE—if 100 women are in a rape situation and they do exactly as they have been taught, how many will be successful and how many will fail? Does the particular method have a high success rate against both types of rapists (Type I and Type II), and, is the strategy based on sound principles and fact, and not on emotion and tradition?

We hear story after story of women who have successfully avoided rape. We listen and frequently draw conclusions about avoidance based on what worked for them. It is *very* important to understand that when looking at rape, those who are most likely to talk about the assault and report the crime, are the individuals who successfully avoided the assault. Conspicuously absent from this group of females who talk about the crime, are the females who did not escape the rape.

Keep in mind that over half of the rapists *will not* resort to physical violence. This means that anything an intended victim does to resist will succeed at least half of the time. These females are the most likely to tell someone. The victims who were not able to get away rarely talk to anyone.

Now let's look at some of the avoidance strategies that are in use today.

RELAX AND GO LIMP

As I see it, the first rung on the evolutionary ladder was the "Relax and Go Limp" strategy. Proponents assume three things, the first is that when a woman resists she excites the male. As was pointed out, one thing the rapist needs in the Rape Sequence is to control the female and have her be submissive. How much more submissive can you get than to go limp?!! This plays right into the rapist's plans!!

The second problem with this strategy is, its proponents believe that rape is sexually motivated and by letting the man get on and off, as it were, the woman would not be harmed. It is incredibly insensitive and unrealistic to advise a woman to relax while some male uses her for a receiving station for violence and sexual domination. It is also unbelievable that anyone would think that *no* harm would come to the woman—what about her mind? Though there may be no physical damage, the emotional damage could be tremendous.

The third assumption is that if you submit you will survive. The fact is that only a very small fraction of stranger rapists are killers. In all likelihood you will survive no matter what. If he is a killer, submission will do nothing to break the rape sequence and stop him.

There is no evidence that would give any success rate at all to this strategy. Success means avoiding the assault, not giving in to it!

BLUFFS AND PLOYS

The next strategy involves the teaching of the "Bluffs and Ploys" theory. The proponents of this strategy advise women to say such things as:

- "I was raped as a child!"
- "I have V.D.!"
- "My boyfriend will be right here!"
- "I'm pregnant!"
- "I have A.I.D.S.!"

or attempt to do such things as:

- urinate on him,
- vomit,
- growl like a dog,
- fake an epileptic seizure,
- rock on the floor while singing a silly song,

and many, many other equally ridiculous things! Not only are these techniques dehumanizing to the woman, but they are ignorantly based on a few lucky successes. If the man calls the bluff, or ploy, what do you do next?! Are you going to tell him you were just practicing your acting skills? How long can you fake an epileptic seizure? It is difficult to believe that very many of us can urinate on command in a high stress situation, or vomit at will. The people who advocate this method of avoidance are telling you that you don't have the ability to defeat the rapist, so your only hope is to make yourself disgusting to him.

Such tricks are well known to assailants! Whenever I interview rapists, I ask them about strategies they think women will use against them; "Ploys and Bluffs" are invariably mentioned.

MARTIAL ARTS

The next step on the evolutionary ladder is one that is widely practiced today—"Martial Arts." We are seeing countless females learning Judo, Karate, and other martial arts with the assumption that they are preparing themselves to defeat a male in an assault situation. Though the success rate of *highly skilled* martial arts practitioners is relatively high, there are very few people who can stay with the training long enough to develop the skill necessary to defeat most rapists in a realistic street situation.

The dynamics of a rape are generally much different than anything martial arts instructors know and teach. The only real positive, short term result which comes from studying martial arts, is the student generally carries herself more confidently. This alone could prevent her from being selected as a target. The bottom line, however, is that unless a woman receives extensive martial arts training specific to rape situations, she will have about the same chance to defeat a rapist as a female not educated in the arts.

SELF-DEFENSE—FIGHT BACK

This step is called the "Self-Defense, Fight Back" theory. The proponents of this strategy advise females to give immediate, vigorous resistance by yelling, assuming a fighting stance, kicking, striking etc. These students are taught to use techniques which, its teachers say, incapacitate the assailant. This is quite true when used against most Type I assailants. However, for a Type II, the techniques are often ineffective and, in fact, elicit a more violent response from the assailant. When you fight, there are no other options—you either win or lose based on your ability to beat the male!!

Other problems exist with this strategy. First, when human beings are in stress situations several things occur within the body that *mask* pain for a period of time. Rapists think about what they are going to do before they do it—which causes stress. They may not know their victim, but they do know, basically, how they are going to rape. In other words, they are mentally practicing for the assault. This preparation causes adrenalin to be released. Also, medical scientists at Johns Hopkins University have discovered the presence of chemicals called endorphins, produced by our bodies which act as pain killers. These endorphins are released when the body is under stress. A final reaction which occurs within the body involves something called, "pain gates," that block pain messages from being transmitted to the brain and then back to the point of injury.

In other words, if you walk up to a stranger on the street and kick him in the groin, stomp on his foot, punch his nose, etc. he will be incapacitated with pain. *However,* if you were to attempt these techniques against a rapist motivated by violence, he will most likely not feel what you have done to him—the pain will be masked for a period of time. How much damage could he do to a female before adrenalin, endorphins, and pain gates are overridden by pain, causing him to stop? There are, literally, thousands of stories in which people have experienced incredibly painful injuries, yet, were able to function, for a period of time, before being incapacitated by the pain. The problem here is not that most of the techniques don't inflict pain; it is that the pain is not felt for a period of time!

A second major problem with the "Fight Back" strategy is that a lot of the techniques taught, simply do not work. Why? Angles of attack and the mechanics of the body are much different in real situations versus posed, controlled learning situations.

As an example, the knee is one of the most popular areas "experts" say to attack, yet in reality, it seldom incapacitates the rapist. Most victims don't know the male is a rapist until he is within arm's distance from the female making it almost impossible to kick the knee. (Fig. 3.1). Unless he is wearing a sign which says he is a rapist, you just don't know until after he is close to you.

Also, in stressful, fighting situations, such as rape, the male has his knees bent. The amount of force needed to incapacitate the male through damaging his knee is beyond the ability of all but the most

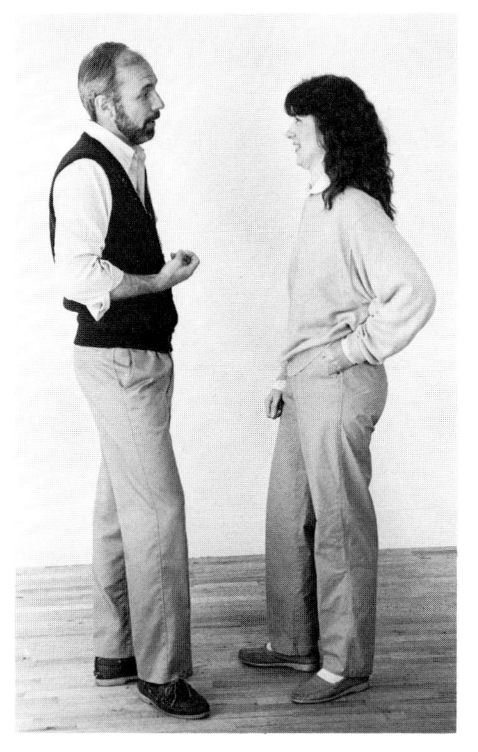

Figure 3.1 ■ Male close to female.

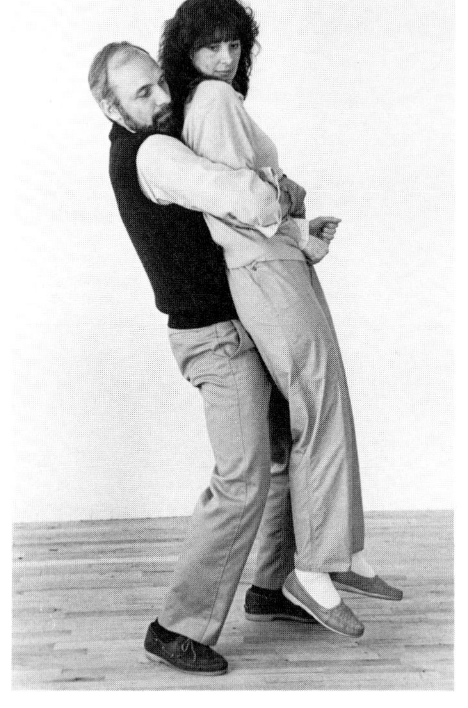

Figure 3.2 ■ Picking up.

skilled and powerful. This holds true if the male attacks from behind by picking the female up or by choking her. (Fig. 3.2, Fig. 3.3). His knees are bent and it is virtually impossible to hurt them!!!

Experts also advise females to try, if being choked from the front, (Fig. 3.4) to knock the man's arms out and then strike him somewhere. This *does not work!* The man is angry and his arms are bent. It takes far more force than you or I could generate to break the grip. Also, unless you are a cone-head, his hands would be forced up under your chin.

There are many other equally ineffective techniques that are taught. The bottom line is there are many stories of successes, but what must be considered is how many times will these techniques work if used against 100 different rapists? What happens to the woman when, and if, it doesn't work?

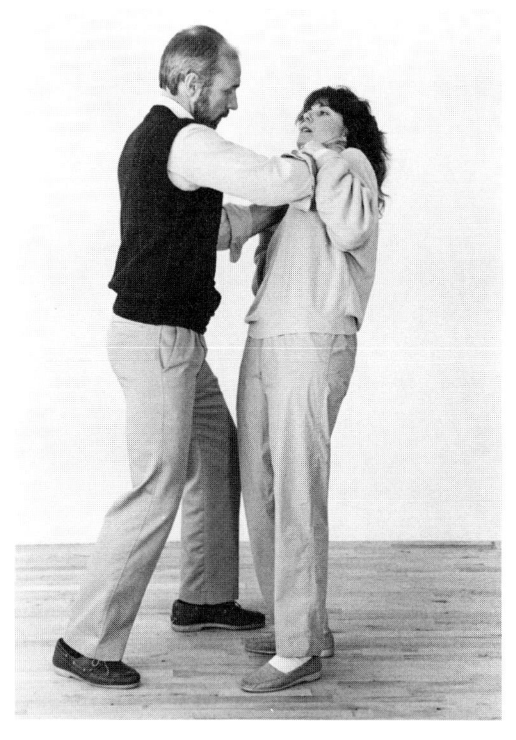

Figure 3.3 ■ Choking.

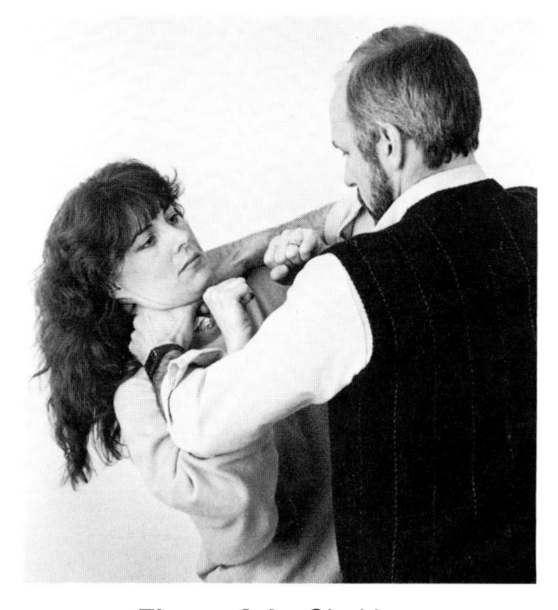

Figure 3.4 ■ Choking.

WEAPONS

The use of weapons to confront the rapist is advocated by many people. There are three questions you must ask yourself when thinking about using a weapon: Is it with you and readily accessible at all times? Do you know how to use it and have you practiced? Will the weapon completely incapacitate all rapists? Unless the answer is yes to all three, the effectiveness will not be much more than 50–50.

Before examining weapons individually, there are a few problems that relate to all weapons.

- Weapons tend to give people a false sense of security. This can cause them to put themselves into situations they normally would not go into. As an example, many women carrying chemical sprays have been targeted and raped by males while walking by themselves in a dark, deserted environment. It is doubtful that the females would have been so vulnerable had they not had the spray.

- I have found that in a good percentage of attacks, the female does not have her weapon in position and ready to use. How many females answer the door to their residence with a chemical spray, knife, or gun in their hand? Yet approximately 50 percent of all sexual assaults occur in the home. Also, because most assaults begin with a testing stage, females are not generally prepared for the situation escalating from talk to violence.

- Few females train themselves in the use of a weapon. Many people have a preconceived notion of a victory, simply because they have a weapon. I have interviewed many females who said they had a weapon, such as a gun, yet did not ever practice with it or even know how to load it.

- Emphasizing weapons denies the fact that the body is your best weapon. It places the responsibility of protection on an inanimate object, such as a key, instead of using the body's ability to protect itself.

Now, let's examine the most popular weapons as they relate to sexual assault avoidance.

Car or House Keys. Without a doubt these are the second most used weapon today. Females are told to arrange them between their fingers and when attacked, jab them into the male's face. (Fig. 3.5.)

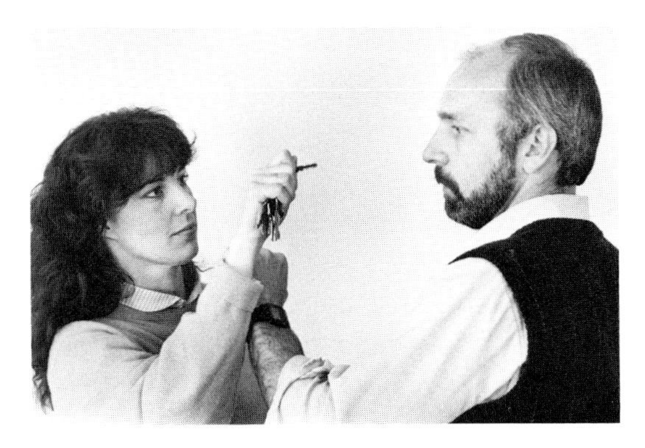

Figure 3.5 ■ Picture of keys in hand.

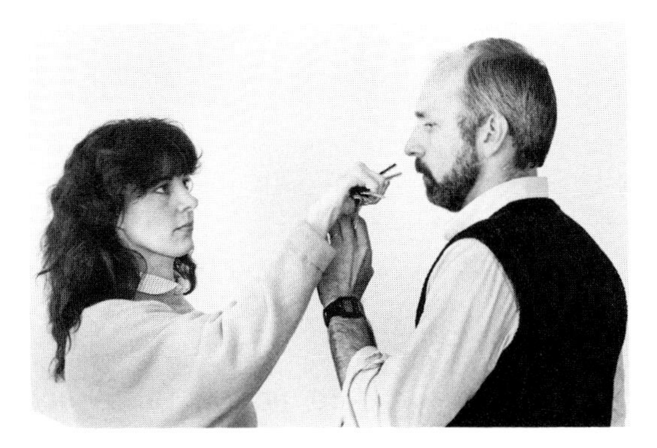

Figure 3.6 ■ Two keys in hand.

It's difficult to understand how a rational person who sets him or herself up as an expert, can say that keys (Fig. 3.6), are a better weapon than your own fingers! If you were going to jab at the eyes (I discourage this), doesn't it stand to reason that these:

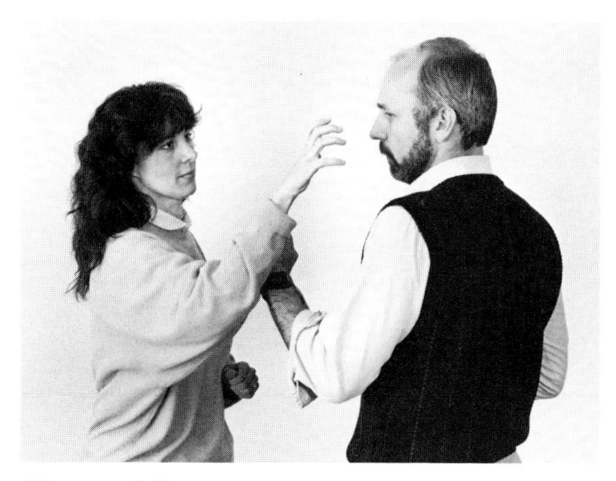

Figure 3.7 ▪ Picture of extended fingers.

would have a much better chance than these:

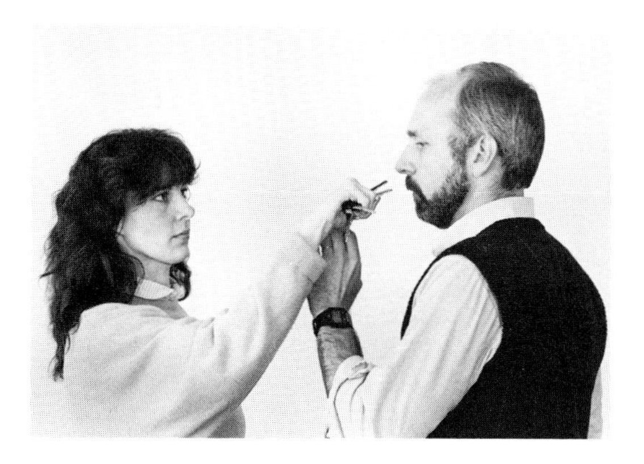

Figure 3.8 ▪ Picture of keys.

You always have your hands with you, and it is unnecessary to look through pockets or a purse for them. They are longer, you have more of them, and if you miss, you can quickly compensate.

Chemical Sprays. I believe that sprays have their place (as a deterrent to a Type I and dogs when jogging), but as a weapon to be used against a violent assault, their effectiveness is vastly overrated. There have been several studies done regarding the effectiveness of sprays. It was found that the effects varied depending on the alcohol content in the male's body, the presence of aggression, and on the environment where the spray is used. In the State of Washington, the spray was put directly into the eyes of several volunteers. There were a variety of responses ranging from minimal to extreme distress.

A flight attendant in Los Angeles was walking to her car one night after a flight. She had her spray in her hand with the safety unlocked. A van stopped, the sliding door opened, and a male grabbed her. She sprayed the male, but due to the wind, alcohol, and individual susceptibility, the man was unaffected. He took the spray from her and sprayed it down her throat. She then was hauled into the van and brutally raped.

The basic problem with the spray is, how will it affect your particular assailant? If he is a Type I, he will leave. A Type II—? If it doesn't completely incapacitate him, the male will remain able to attack—an attack that has now become a response to your attempt to defend yourself. Your aggression will generally elicit an extremely violent response.

Knife. Once again, as is the case with all weapons, knowledge in the use of the knife, practice, and accessibility to the weapon are paramount for success. Type I assailants will generally leave at the sight of a weapon. Unfortunately, you cannot know ahead of time if the male is a Type I or II. I have interviewed several rapists who had women use knives against them. The males, with one exception, had no trouble getting the knife from the women. The exception was stabbed but later stated that he'd felt nothing. He got the knife away from her and stabbed the female with it over 25 times.

My mother used to carry a small 1 1/2 inch pen knife. She said, "Don't worry, honey. I can use this to protect myself." After I, myself, ambushed her several times, she realized the futility of carrying such a weapon.

Gun. Handguns are not legal to carry in most states. They have, however, been much more successful than knives. The basic problem with a handgun, is that when you need to use it you do not have it in hand. Few rapists break into a residence—the female opens the door to him. Because of this, even if she did have a gun, she could not be prepared to use it. Also, special training, with a lot of practice, is necessary in order to be proficient. The caliber of the gun is very important, as it relates to Knock-Down Potential. The lower the potential, the less success. A gun with a 22 caliber would have questionable effect on a Type II at close range—the effect of a 45 caliber gun is less doubtful. If you are going to have a gun in your home for protection, I suggest that it be a shotgun. Skill in aiming is not necessary, and the Knock-Down Potential is high.

Undoubtedly, there are many other weapons females have been advised to use. It is very important to note that almost any weapon you can imagine has had some success. The idea we must always keep in mind is its *success rate*. How many times has it succeeded versus how many failures? There is no weapon—none—that can equal the success of the techniques you will be given in the fourth 'C'.

The major problem with any confrontational strategy is, if you fail, what do you do? There is no backup! Once you start fighting, you either win or lose based on your ability to fight an opponent who is, generally, of greater size, strength, and has more fighting experience.

■ ■ ■ ■

The final step in the evolutionary ladder, as I see it, is the Four 'C's'. This system gives females alternatives to being a victim and is based on a progressive system of workable choices; choices that take into account the two types of sexual assailants. The beauty of this system is its simplicity. It will make sense to you, it's easy to use, and is the most successful strategy of sexual assault avoidance available.

FOUR "C's" OVERVIEW

Now that you are aware of the rape sequence and the evolution of sexual assault avoidance strategies, let's briefly examine how the Four 'C's' can interrupt the sequence. Remember, the first step the rapist takes, is to find a vulnerable female.

Your first 'C'—Concern for Personal Safety—is designed to prevent the possibility of you being selected as a target. By reducing your vulnerability, you drastically lower the chances that you will be assaulted.

If, however, you are confronted by a possible sexual assailant, 'C' #2—Confidence and 'C' #3—Control—will, most often, prevent the male from succeeding in his attempts to have you test out positively. You will learn how to control the situation so that you do not show the necessary submissive signals he needs in order to carry the sequence into its next step. It must be understood that most sexual assaults do not start with violent aggressive behavior. The "experts" who are preparing women to assume a fighting stance, jam keys in the eyes, etc., are undoubtedly unaware of this fact or choose to ignore it. If the female is equipped with the proper psychological weapons, she can often defeat the male before aggression and violence enter the situation.

Unfortunately, there are times when the rapist skips over the second step in the rape sequence and moves right into the aggressive stage of intimidation. If this is the case, 'C' #3 can still afford you a good chance of getting out of the situation.

However, if the psychological approach is failing, or you are not given the chance to use it, 'C' #4—Complete Incapacitation—can be utilized to defeat the assailant. The techniques you will be shown are 100 percent effective. They will be easy to learn and use—they will completely incapacitate the male!

To summarize, it must be strongly emphasized that there are really two distinct types of sexual assailants: Type I—Sexual Confrontation, and Type II—Violent Sexual Attack. To be effective, a system of assault avoidance must not only be able to defeat both types, but must also be based upon knowledge of the rape sequence and on an awareness of how to use sound principles in order to interrupt the sequence.

CHAPTER

4

Concern for Personal Safety—Your First 'C'

The goal of 'C' #1 is to counter the rapist's attempts at selecting you as a target. Remember, this selection process is based upon the rapist's perceptions of the vulnerability of the victim. When you reduce your vulnerability, you greatly reduce the chances of being targeted as a victim.

This option is not intended to, nor will it, restrict your life. It is not called, "Do's and Don'ts," "Rules to Live By," or any number of other equally restrictive and insulting names. The basic idea is for you to look at your particular lifestyle and limit your vulnerability where possible. For example, let's say you enjoy jogging. There are many who would say *only* run during the day with other people. What if your job doesn't allow it? Are you supposed to give up something you enjoy? I don't believe that should be the case and I doubt if you do either. To limit your vulnerability in this situation, you could attempt to find someone who could run with you at night, run in a residential area, run or walk against traffic, attempt to stay in well lighted areas, or run at an indoor track. If none of these ideas suits you, run anyway. Adapt this 'C' to you!!

It would be unrealistic to believe that all measures to limit vulnerability could be taken at all times. If you find that there are instances when it is extremely inconvenient to use them, do not worry about it. Simply be more alert—you will learn in following chapters what to do if you are selected as a target.

The following are measures suggested to limit your vulnerability. They will be broken down into specific areas of vulnerability. For the most part, these measures can, and should, be used by males as well. Though the crime may differ, we can all be victims!

RESIDENCE OR EXTENSION OF (MOTEL, HOTEL, COLLEGE DORM)

Approximately 50 percent of all sexual assaults take place in the female's place of residence—the place where she should be able to feel safest. I have found that the rapist seldom breaks in. In a majority of cases, the victim has willingly opened the door to the male. Because of this it is important to be aware of several measures which will help to limit your vulnerability.

Answering the Door

By posing as delivery persons, salespersons, maintenance personnel, utility workers, or using a variety of other disguises, many rapists are able to gain access without force. When answering the door to someone like this, we tend to believe they are as they represent themselves. We either do not want to be embarrassed by mistrusting them or we know no other alternative. Additionally, most of us do not believe that we will ever be victims. Rapists know this and they use it to their advantage.

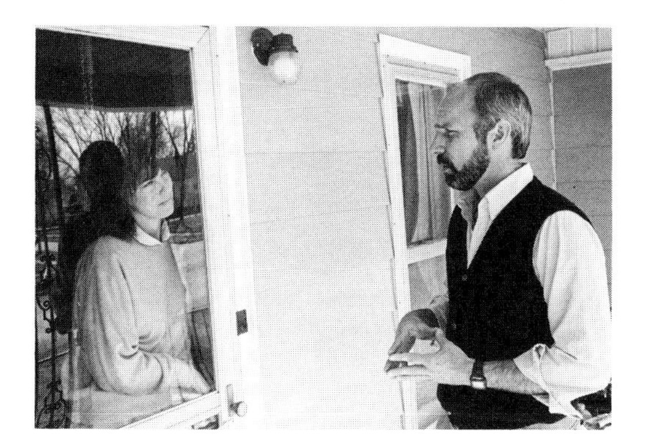

Figure 4.1 ■ Woman talking to a man from behind screen or storm door.

As an experiment for my classes, I had two of my students select seven homes or apartments in the community. Accompanying me in my jeep, we went to each of these residences. Posing as a United Parcel Service delivery person, clad in jeans, tennis shoes, baseball cap, and carrying a clipboard and package, I proceeded to knock on the doors of each home. Each time, it was answered by a female who allowed me in when I asked her to sign for the package. None of the females asked to see my identification or questioned why I drove a jeep to deliver the packages. After gaining entrance into their homes, I eventually revealed my identity and we then discussed measures for reducing their vulnerability.

It is incredible how believable rapists can be!! *Verifying* that people are who they say they are is *essential.* If you own a home that has a secure storm or screen door, keep it locked and talk with the male from behind the secured door (Fig. 4.1). If you are an apartment dweller, try to have a peep hole in the door, and/or, if possible, a mail slot (Fig. 4.2). The cost of these items is under $30, but the peace of mind they offer is priceless.

When an unfamiliar male comes to your door and asks for entry for *any* reason, verify he is who he claims to be by requiring him to present identification. He should either hold it up so you can see it through the peep hole, pass it through the mail slot, or simply show it to you through the screen or storm door. If you are not satisfied, take his name, company, and any other pertinent information and call his

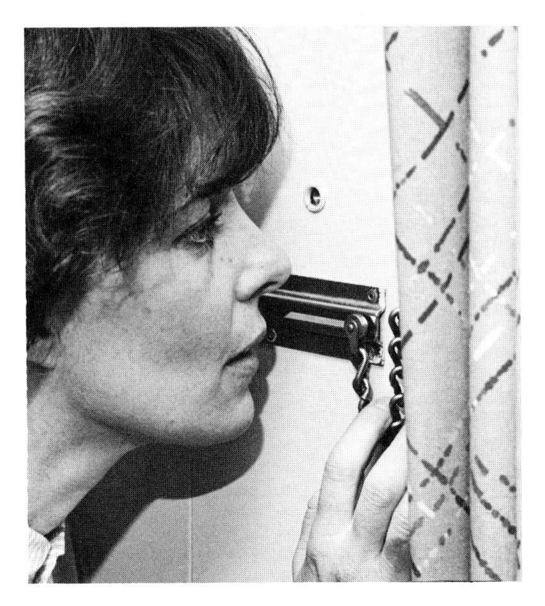

Figure 4.2 ■ Door with peep hole and mail slot.

employer to verify. If the male refuses, or he is not who he says, immediately call the police.

Allow no one access to you unless:

- You know and trust them.
- You are expecting them.
- You have verified they are who they say they are, and you want them to enter.

Developing a sense of self, and not being concerned with what a stranger may think of you, is essential to becoming less vulnerable. In situations like this, rapists hope you will trust them and thus present yourself as a target.

Apartment Hunting

As a consumer, when you shop for an apartment there are certain factors that make one apartment more secure than another. Things to look for:

- second floor and above provide more security and privacy.
- a main entrance that is well lighted, locked, and/or guarded.
- lighted and secure parking facilities within the building grounds.
- dead-bolt door locks.
- intercom and/or peep hole.
- mail slot.
- knowledge of, and a confident feeling about, the people who occupy apartments around yours.

Summary

By keeping your doors and windows secured, and not allowing males into your residence whom you do not know and have not verified through identification, you virtually eliminate one of the most successful methods rapists use to target a victim. Think of yourself first and do not worry about the attitudes of a stranger at your door.

Parking Lots

Sexual assaults that occur outside of the female's residence are most often directed against a solitary female in an environment where there is little chance for support.

The most common method strangers use to Select and Approach/Test outside of the home is this. The rapist will observe a parking lot. It could be outside of *any* retail establishment or company. As the woman leaves the building, the male approaches her and verbally disarms her by politely asking a few questions. If she stops to talk with him, he will continue to be nice and talk, while at the same time moving closer. If/when he feels the timing is right, i.e. no one around, he escalates.

How do you break this particular method of assaulting? First, try to avoid situations such as these where you or I would be vulnerable due to the time of day. It is easier to avoid a situation than it is to get out of one.

Second, if you are in an environment that gives you little chance for support, and someone approaches you, give a brief assertive answer to his question while continuing to go to your car. Do not stop, and do not apologize for it. Expect that he will try to talk with you further. Be firm by saying, "I am in a hurry, good night!" Usually this will break the sequence due to the fact that he is not able to control you. The sad reality is that someone else will soon come along who will stop.

At Work

Many females have jobs which demand late hours. When they leave their workplace, they are often alone in a deserted environment. If this is the case. there are a few steps that can be taken to greatly reduce vulnerability.

- Park as close to your workplace as possible, preferably in an area that is lighted and guarded.

- If you have a choice, take the work home instead of staying alone in the building.

- When you leave the building, be aware of your surroundings and walk briskly, and confidently to your car.

- If you are uneasy about going to your car alone, and there are security personnel present, ask them to either escort you, or watch as you go to your car.

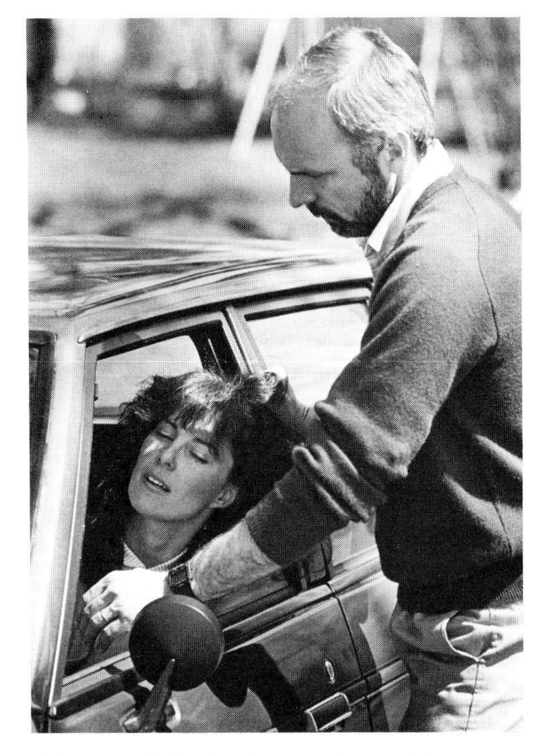

Figure 4.3 ▪ Male reaching into car.

Car Travel

In the last few years the number of assaults on women in their cars has risen at a phenomenal rate. There are several measures that may be taken to limit vulnerability while traveling by car.

Always try to remember to keep your doors locked, and your windows rolled up enough to prevent a hand from reaching in when you are stopped for lights or signs (Fig. 4.3).

If you are in a minor accident and the environment is such that you would feel vulnerable if you left your car (i.e., dark, deserted street, male, or males in the other vehicle), stay in your car. Compare licenses and insurance companies through a small opening in your window (Fig. 4.5). A very popular ploy used by rapists is to target a female alone in her car. When she is at a stop the male bumps into her car. When she gets out to assess the damage she is threatened and generally forced into the car and raped (Fig. 4.4). Unless you

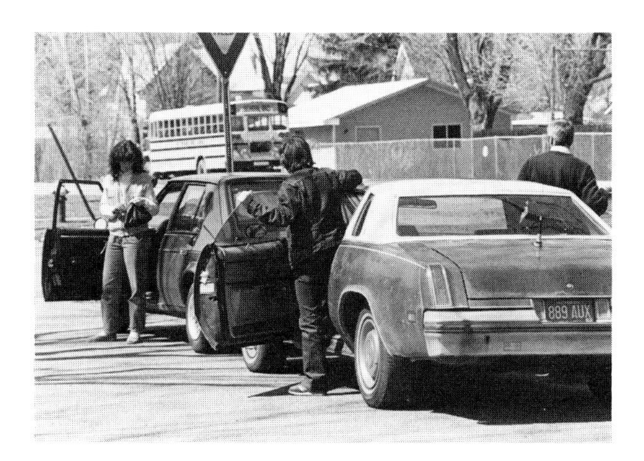

Figure 4.4 ■ Comparing drivers licenses. Female's car was hit.

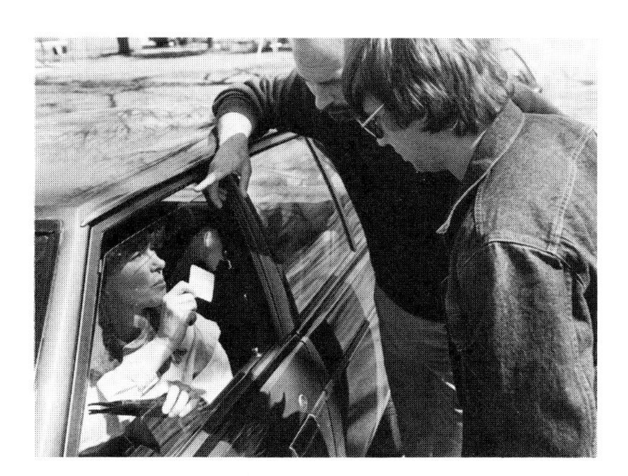

Figure 4.5 ■ Correct way with window up and inside the car.

are in an environment that is safe, and the accident is obviously not a ploy, do not get out of your car until the police arrive. If you do not think that the police will be coming to the scene, advise the person who hit your car that you are going to a service station, etc. to call.

When traveling outside of town, attempt to use well traveled roads. A female traveling on a secluded road is seen as being very vulnerable.

If you have a breakdown while out of town, raise the hood and stay inside your car with the doors locked. If a male stops and offers help, talk to him from inside your car. Under no circumstance allow

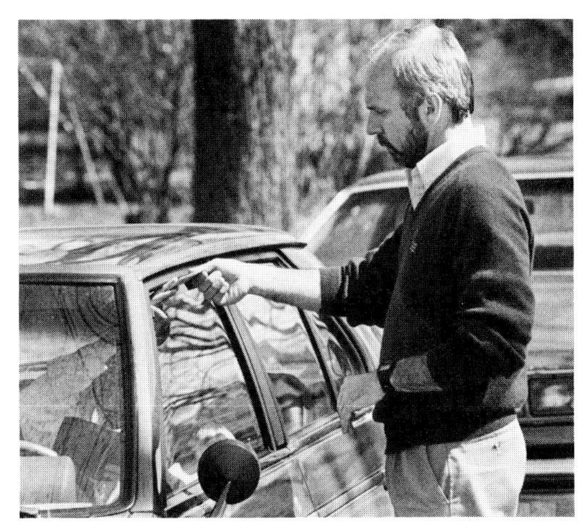

Figure 4.6 ■ Showing female getting information through window.

him into your car. After all, it is your car—a male cannot pump the accelerator and turn the key any better than you. If, by looking under the hood, he cannot locate and fix the problem, ask him to go to the nearest service station and send back assistance. If you find that the situation necessitates that you go with him, there are a few procedures to follow:

- Always be sure you have a spare key to your car and residence hidden in your purse or wallet.
- Keep a pad of paper and pencil in your glove compartment.
- On the pad of paper, write the make of car you will be leaving in, license plate number, the man's name and driver's license number, and the time you expect to arrive at your residence (Fig. 4.6).
- Display this on the dash.
- Leave your keys in the ignition and exit you car on the side opposite the male (Fig. 4.7).

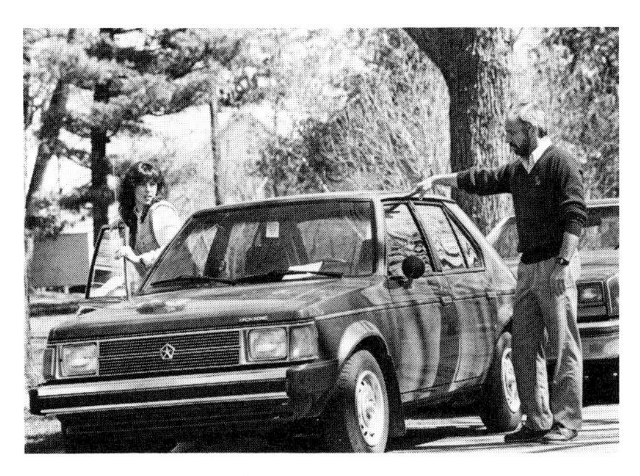

Figure 4.7 ▪ Getting out of vehicle opposite of where male is.

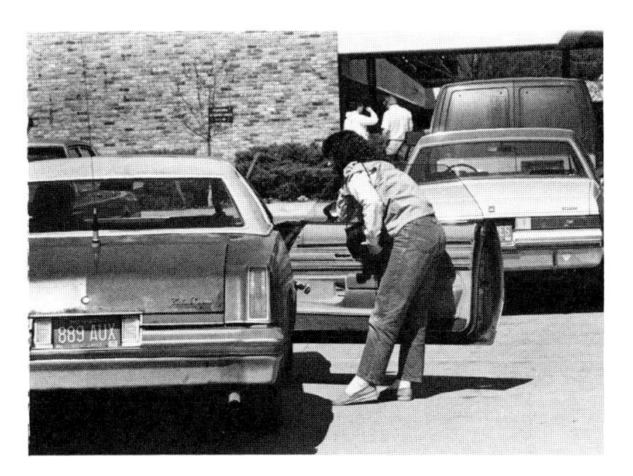

Figure 4.8 ▪ Being dropped off.

- Quickly close the locked door and make a fuss about the fact that you locked your keys in the car

Why do all of this? By locking your keys in the car you prevent the male from taking the keys from you, unlocking the door, and destroying the paper with his name, etc. Have the male either drop you off at your residence, a friend's, or some lighted place with a phone so you can call someone (Fig. 4.8). When you get to your residence you will have an extra key to unlock the door. The next day, or whenever, you can go back to your car with help.

If this procedure is not followed, and the male is a rapist, there will be absolutely no record or evidence of your whereabouts. Following this procedure limits your vulnerability and shows you not to be submissive.

Another common way of targeting a female in her car is for the rapist to pose as a police officer. He is most often dressed in plain clothes, driving a car that does not appear to be a police car. The revolving light on the top of the car, or on the dash makes his victim think he is an officer.

This type of assault generally occurs at night in a location that will attract little attention. You see the flashing lights in your mirror and pull over. The man will walk up to the car and use one of two techniques to get you to step out. First, he may say something such as; "I am off-duty and I'm sorry I had to stop you but both your tail lights are out. This is really a hazard. If you wouldn't mind getting out of the car to verify, I can sign a form that will give you 48 hours to correct the problem." He is very nice and always has a believable reason for stopping you.

The second tactic is to be much more aggressive with you. He may be dressed like an officer, but most likely will still be in plain clothes. He will try to get you out of the car by telling you he has to search it, or give you a sobriety test. He may threaten you—"Get out, get out now or I'll have to arrest you." This can be very intimidating.

What should you do if stopped for no apparent reason?

- Keep your door locked. Slightly open the window to verify his credentials. Look closely at the badge or I.D.

- When you are in a location where there are few people, do not get out of the car. Be polite and either ask that another officer be called in or, ask to go to an area that is well lit with people around.

- If he physically threatens, drive to a police station, or any other area where there would be support for you. Be quick—do not be concerned about him.

Law enforcement officers are well aware of these methods of targeting. If you are polite and assertive, few real officers would be upset by your distrust. Verify and trust your instincts!

Summary

When outside of your home, be alert to situations where you may be vulnerable. If you cannot limit your vulnerability do not worry, just "tune" into your environment and remember that you have other options. Regardless of where you are, always attempt to show yourself as confident and assertive, not submissive. Body language is important—be aware of what you are showing!

THE FEMALE FLYER

Throughout the world today, more than ever before, females are travelling by themselves on business and pleasure. Going from airport to airport and hotel to hotel, puts females in situations of high vulnerability. To limit the vulnerability and make travel safer, the following procedures could be employed.

Prior to Your Trip

Be sure that your residence is securely locked. Try to have a neighbor or the police watch your residence for you.

If parking at the airport, attempt to park as close to the entrance as possible. A lighted area would be preferred. Make sure your doors and windows are locked.

Walk briskly and confidently to the terminal. Slow moving, submissive looking females, are often selected as targets by males who cruise parking facilities.

It is best to schedule your flights so that you are using the airport when there are many travelers present. Deserted airport terminals have been the scene for many assaults.

Transportation to Hotel or Appointment

Most reputable hotels will have a *marked* limousine service available to guests. Some hotels have the service on demand, which necessitates calling and asking for the limousine to be sent. If the vehicle is unmarked, ask the name of the driver, then verify. Other hotels have a set schedule for guest pickup. Whichever system is used, wait inside the terminal or with a group. A solitary figure standing next to the street is very vulnerable.

When using a taxi service, attempt to stick with well known companies. When in doubt, ask an airline sky cap located outside most terminal buildings to recommend a cab company.

Whether using a limousine service or taxi, make sure that the driver lets you out as close to the hotel or building entrance as possible.

At the Hotel

Safety at hotels and motels is something with which everyone should be concerned. This is a prime area for assault and robbery.

When checking into the hotel, the desk clerk should not shout your room number. If he or she does this, caution him or her and ask for another room. Rapists have waited in hotel lobbies and overheard the room number and name of the female she checked in. The male then locates the room and poses as an employee to gain entrance. Sometimes they will intercept the female just as she has unlocked her door and is about to enter her room. (Fig. 4.9)

Most hotels will provide you with a bellman or escort to your room if you request it. If this service is not available, use caution. Do not hesitate to leave the elevator or hallway if you have an uncomfortable feeling about someone in either. Have your key ready! If there is a male near your room, or approaching it, wait to open your door until he is far enough away that he could not rush into your room before you have a chance to secure the door.

Once you are in your room, check all doors and windows to make sure they can be securely locked. If they cannot, ask for another room. It is advisable to ask for rooms above the second floor so that the windows and/or balcony will be more secure.

As was previously mentioned, hotel rape is often accomplished by a male who poses as an employee of the hotel. He may come to your door and announce that he has a complimentary basket of fruit. He may say that he is with hotel maintenance and must check something such as the TV or air-conditioning. He may say he is with

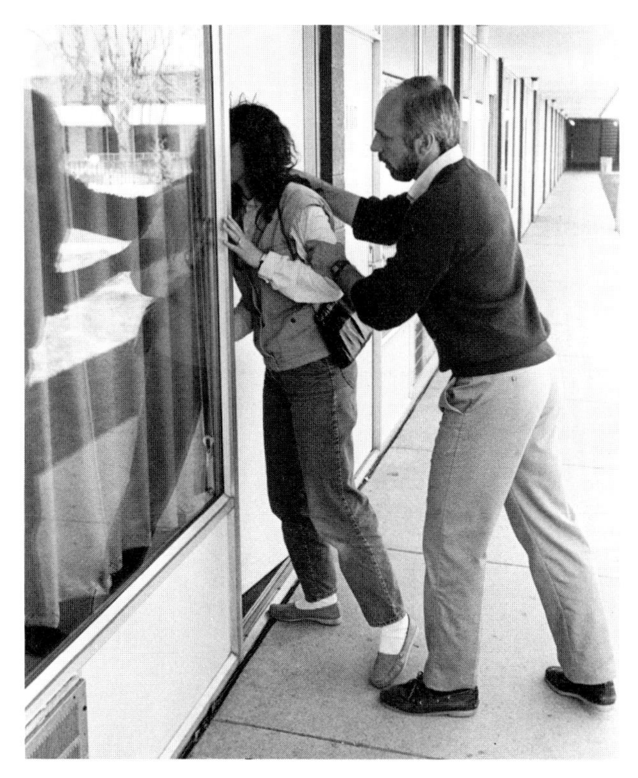

Figure 4.9

housekeeping or any number of other creative ploys. Once again, unlock you door to no one until the credentials have been verified. To do this, simply get the male's name and responsibility, and call the front desk to verify.

If you eat at the hotel or go to the lounge for a drink, be alert to males attempting to test you. Do not hesitate to be assertive and tell a male you are not interested. If you feel someone is attempting to follow you to your room, or if you are being hassled by someone, seek assistance from an employee of the hotel.

Trip's End

When scheduling your trip, attempt to schedule so you will be returning during daylight hours. Observe the path you must take to reach your car and the area surrounding you car. You are looking for anything which is suspicious. A male fumbling with his keys, checking his tires, watching you, etc. If you feel uncomfortable, move away and observe. Seek assistance from airport security if necessary.

Walk briskly and confidently to your car. Once inside, lock your doors and keep the windows up until you are out of the parking facility.

When you reach your residence check it for anything out of the ordinary, such as a door or window ajar, marks by the lock, etc. If there is something which arouses your suspicion, do not go in—call the police.

Summary

The female flyer, though vulnerable, can greatly reduce her risk by using these simple procedures and by showing herself to be confident and assertive. Do not hesitate to seek assistance if you feel you need it. Above all else, do not worry about embarrassing yourself or others by asking for verification of credentials, for another room, or for anything else. You are the most important person there!!!

THE SOCIAL SCENE

Another area that merits mentioning has to do with being vulnerable to strangers in social settings. Quite often a rapist will target a female in a bar, at a party, etc. and attempt to determine if she can be subtly controlled. Generally, if he can dominate and control he will attempt to set her up in an environment where there is no support,—maybe by offering to take her home, to another social setting, etc. Once in the environment in which she is more vulnerable, he becomes more aggressive and then. . . .

Actually, this is a scene played nightly in almost every bar. The difference is, a normal male may become more aggressive but if the female does not respond positively, he will stop; frustrated maybe, but he will stop. However, a rapist will not stop.

What can you do to limit your vulnerability and yet still meet people? Primarily, be assertive and qualify the male. what I mean by this is don't let him dominate and control you, the conversation, etc. Talk with him and make him talk. If you find that you would like to spend more time with him, do it, but on your terms. Maybe you could meet him on "neutral turf" a time or two. Once you feel comfortable with him, then do what pleases you. Most rapists are not patient enough to spend time on two or more separate occasions testing. There are too many people out there who are more vulnerable. If you have misjudged, don't worry—you have options.

THE "NICE GUY"

A final area that is of concern, has to do with avoiding being targeted by a "Nice Guy." It is important that you remember who he is and how he operates. He will look for a target he knows, be nice, and probably very attentive. He will work towards creating a situation where he is alone with her.

Following are a few suggestions to avoid this type of situation.

- Be assertive. If someone says or does *anything* that makes you uncomfortable, confront their behavior and/or avoid them.

- Be sure you know your limits and where alcohol is concerned. If a man attempts to get you to drink more than you are comfortable with, say no! Expect some pressure.

- Until you really feel you can trust this person, do things on your terms. See him for lunch. Have him come to your place when friends are around. Drive your own car. Keep to situations where you are not isolated with him. If he is truly a good man, he will not be upset by this.

Just because you are familiar with someone does not mean they are worthy of your trust. You owe no one anything! If you feel uncomfortable or pressured, take action. Do not ignore your instincts.

SUMMARY OF 'C' #1—CONCERN FOR PERSONAL SAFETY

Altruism, sacrificing your feelings and well-being for another, is the nemesis of us all. The key to limiting vulnerability, is to monitor your lifestyle and environment and avoid potentially vulnerable situations where possible. Be concerned with yourself *first,* and do not concern yourself at all with what others may think when your safety is at stake or in jeopardy.

If, in spite of your attempts to limit vulnerability, you find yourself a potential target, move to the next two 'C's.

Chapter 4 Worksheet

Look at your lifestyle (work, transportation, recreation, socialization, etc.) and list those times when you are most vulnerable.

Under each one, list what you could do to limit your vulnerability. Be realistic!!

CHAPTER

5

CONFIDENCE AND CONTROL—YOUR SECOND AND THIRD 'C'S'

In very basic terms, these two 'C's' involve taking command of the situation and manipulating the male until you can get away from him or around people. Because most sexual assaults begin with talking, knowing *what* to say and *how* to say it can eliminate the conflict before it progresses to a point where the man attempts to harm you.

Today, most females are being told to "fight back, don't allow the male near you, teach him a lesson," etc., etc. As I stated in a previous chapter, if the male is nonviolent (Type I), this strategy will most often be successful. However, if the male is potentially a violent person (Type II), the strategy of confrontation often ends with the female extremely battered or worse. Fighting first gives you no other option should it fail!! With all but the Type I, aggression breeds aggression. If you use these

'C's' first, you have a great chance for success. If unsuccessful, you always have the use of the final 'C,' which has never failed.

The principles of Confidence and Control are designed to counter the stages of the rape sequence where the male tests and intimidates his potential victim. His goal is to elicit submissive responses and to dominate the female. In talking with rapists, I have found that they all mentally rehearse the rape prior to actually targeting a woman. That is, they may not know the victim, but they can picture the assault and what they expect will happen. During his rehearsal the Type I pictures the female being intimated, afraid, and nonresistive. The Type II figures she will be intimated and not resist, or she will fight back. He is prepared for either. They *all* expect *Fight* or *Fright*. No rapist expects that the female will love the fact that he is going to rape her.

The reason these work so well, is that you take control of the situation without fighting or showing fright. You psychologically throw the man off balance because you do not act the way he expects you to. Showing confidence, you take control, force him to react to you, and manipulate the situation until you are away from the man or around people. Once around people, you can do whatever you want. If you show yourself as being in control, confident, and not submissive, the male will generally not move into the next step of the rape sequence. The beauty of using these 'C's', is that they will get you away from the male and out of the rape sequence most of the time. If they do not, you can be sure that you are dealing with a Type II, and the use of your fourth 'C' will be appropriate and successful.

PRINCIPLES OF CONFIDENCE

You want to project an image of confidence without attempting to intimidate. The male is looking for a female he can dominate. Appearing confident limits your targetability, and reduces the chance of a male finding success with the Approach/Test Stage of the rape sequence. Rapists generally avoid confident acting females for two specific reasons. First, rapists I have spoken with think that a woman who looks and talks confidently, is much more likely to fight them. The second reason is rapists think that a confident person is much more likely to report an assault. Though neither reason is true, this explains why acting confident and assertive when in a vulnerable situation, will do much to avoid targeting.

Confidence to the point of intimidation, however, calls for a response from the male—he will either allow himself to be intimidated and back off (Type I), or he will feel forced into further action (Type II). This is not a choice you want the male to have to make. Remember, assertiveness not submissiveness!

PRINCIPLES OF CONTROL

Act—Force the Male to React to You

In all rape situations I have studied, the male attempts to control the woman by making her react to his questions or actions. Utilizing this principle, you turn the tables on the rapist and gain control by taking actions which force him to react to you. This is the most critical principle because if you can control him and thus, the situation, you are most likely going to break out of the rape sequence. You ask questions, make statements, and take action designed to get him to respond to you.

Manipulate

The second principle, is to manipulate the situation so that you and the male are moving to a place where you can be safe. This generally means an environment where there are people, such as hotels, lounges, convenience stores, etc. This reduces your vulnerability, and thus decreases the chance that the male will resort to violence to achieve his goal. You move from a place of his choosing, to neutral or safe turf. Once on the safe turf, you can scream, hit, or simply confront the person with his behavior. Be sure there are people around who will support you if you choose to confront the male!!

Humanize

The final broad principle is to show yourself as being a human being, not an object. Rapists interviewed often talk of needing to see their victims as nameless objects, symbols representing something that creates within them the drive to assault. By humanizing, the perspective is changed and, possibly, an advantage is gained for you.

Humanizing is accomplished by giving yourself a name (fictitious or real) and talking about yourself. The important thing is to keep control of the conversation and converse about everyday experiences.

■ ■ ■ ■

The key to the success of this 'C' is that all of these principles are being used *at the same time.* I bet you are saying to yourself, "How can I do this?" Believe me, it is not as hard as it sounds. Look at your day-to-day activities and play the "What if . . . ?" game. You like to jog for instance; practice what you would do if someone attempted to target you while jogging. Don't live in fear either. Plan for the unexpected and mentally rehearse what you do and say if. . . . Picture yourself acting out these 'C's' in different situations that you encounter. What would you say and do that is believable, allows you to control and manipulate the male so that you can get away from him or get somewhere near people. Keep in mind, while rehearsing your acting role, that the male has to see an advantage in going with you. Why would he want to go to an area you choose versus assaulting you right where you are? Why go to a convenience store with you for wine (one means of getting near people) instead of staying in a secluded area?

I believe you will more fully understand how to put these principles into practice when you look at the examples.

PUTTING THE PRINCIPLES INTO PRACTICE

Now that you have the basics, some examples will be given showing the principles being put into practice. All of the examples are factual, and all happened to former students of mine.

In 1975, at a large mid-western university, a student was returning to her resident hall after an evening of research in the library. It was dark and she was

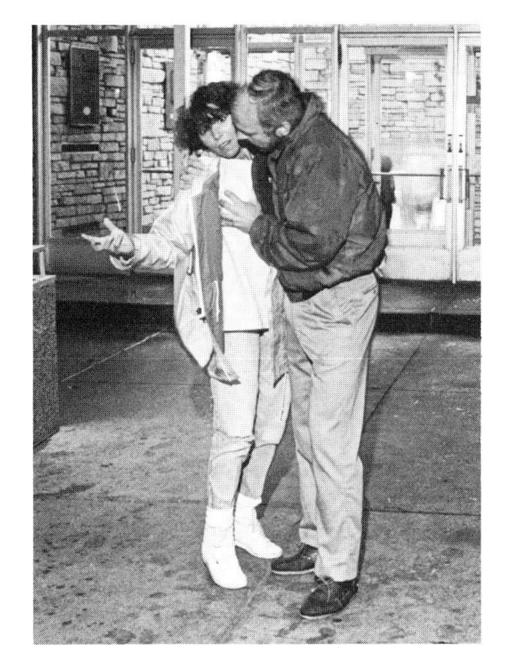

Figure 5.1 ■ Targeting and testing—arm around shoulder.

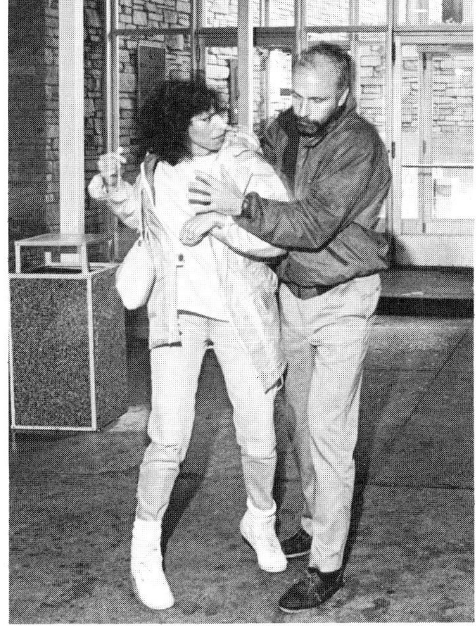

Figure 5.2 ■ Fighting and male about to hit her—WRONG.

alone—vulnerable. A male targeted her and walked up beside her. He began talking with her. Within a minute, he put his arm around her shoulder and brought his hand to rest on her breast (Fig. 5.1). She was shocked, but quickly realized she had two choices: immediately resist by screaming and striking out at him, or attempt to use the psychological principles. The first choice would most always scare a Type I away. Unfortunately, Type II assaults are on the increase, and screaming and striking at a Type II would have undoubtedly elicited a violent response (Fig. 5.2). Realistically, you cannot ask a rapist which type he is before you take action. So, play it safe by treating all potential rapists as Type II's. That way, no painful mistakes will be made.

Visibly shocked, she said, "You're hurting me! I can't believe this is happening. You're not the kind of guy that needs to use these tactics with a woman, are you? There's a better place and time for us to do this. I've had a terrible day and all I want to do is relax. Come on, let's get to know each other first!" This statement did not cause a confrontation, yet it was unexpected and positive. She then told him her name (fictitious) and what she had been doing at the library. At the same time, she took

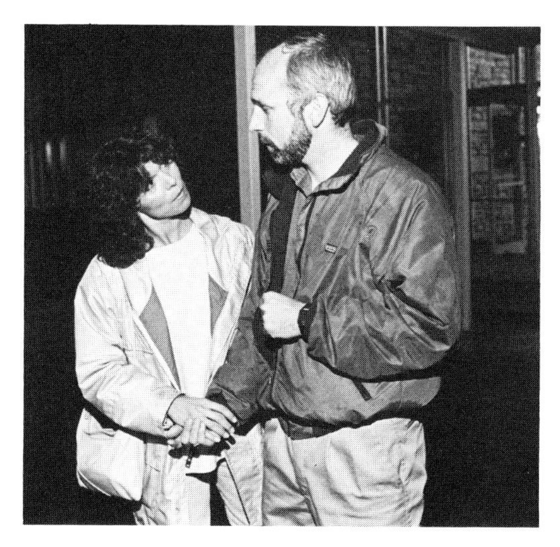

Figure 5.3 ■ Talking and taking his arm—looking confident and controlled.

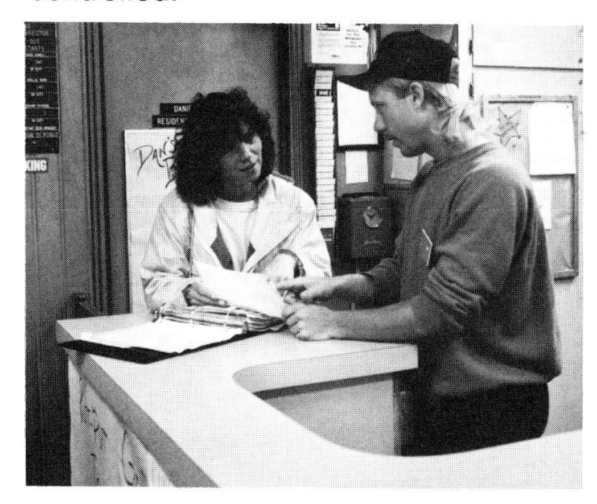

Figure 5.4 ■ Talking to desk clerk.

his arm and started walking toward her residence (Fig. 5.3), and all the while, controlling the situation by talking—never giving the man a chance to focus on his original objective (action, forcing the male to react). Once they entered the residence hall lobby, she excused herself or a minute by telling the male that she had to get some notes to study from the desk clerk. She was very believable and in control of the situation. When she reached the desk she quietly told the clerk to call the police (Fig. 5.4).

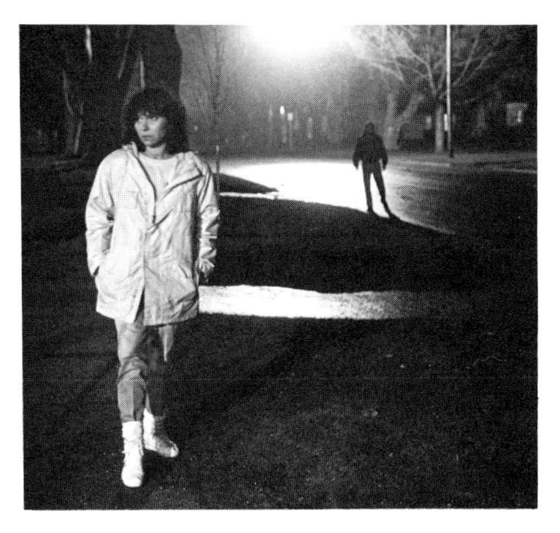

Figure 5.5 ▪ Male approaching.

They arrived just as the male was leaving the lobby. He was charged with sexual assault and convicted.

Remember, if at any time her attempts at taking control failed, she could still have used her body as a weapon. This woman controlled the situation by psychologically throwing the male off balance and by manipulating him to an environment where she would be safe.

Another example happened to a female in an eastern community. The attempted assault was at night in a deserted neighborhood—an ideal targeting environment. This woman was walking from her bus stop to her apartment building. Realizing that she was in a vulnerable situation, she became more aware of her surroundings. Because this was a vulnerable situation she was frequently in, she had played the "What if . . . ?" game to rehearse a course of action if a male ever approached her. As it happened, she began hearing footsteps coming from behind. She increased her pace to determine if she was being pursued, while at the same time, glancing over her shoulder to see who it was (Fig. 5.5) She saw that it was a man and that he was also quickening his pace. Her next action was to look for a place of safety, such as an open grocery store, restaurant, etc. Seeing none, she quickly reviewed, mentally, what she would say and how she would act if, and when, the male got close. When he was ten feet behind her, this woman turned and confidently said, "Hi, thanks for coming up to me!

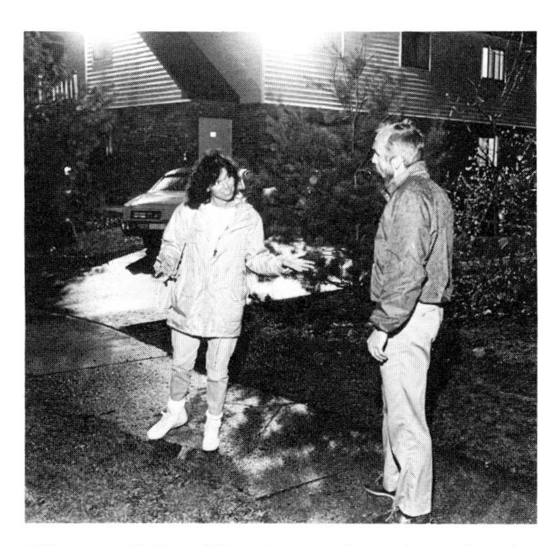

Figure 5.6 ■ She turned and walked up to the male—talking.

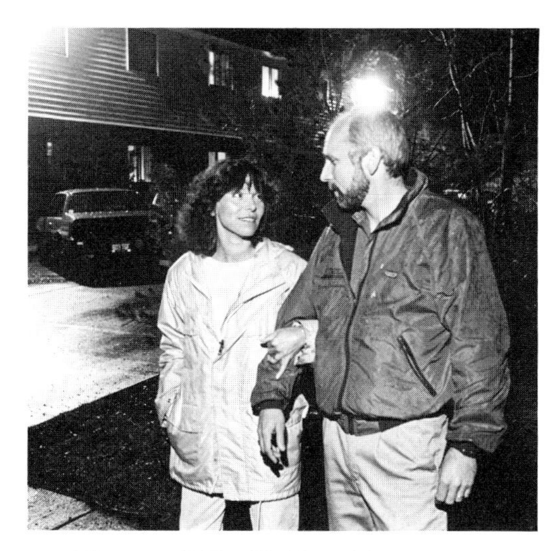

Figure 5.7 ■ Taking his arm.

It is seldom that someone would come up to a perfect stranger and walk with them. I really appreciate the company!'' (Fig. 5.6)

Before allowing the male to answer, she took his arm and began walking at a brisk pace toward her apartment (Fig. 5.7). She did the unexpected—she was not submissive or aggressive. She manipulated the male by showing confidence and controlling the situation. He was

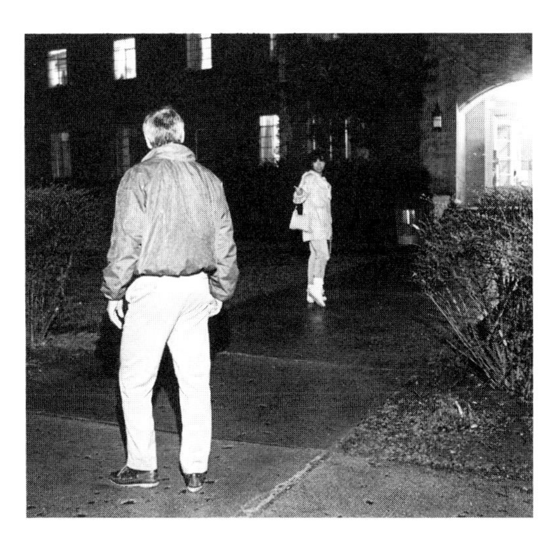

Figure 5.8 ▪ Leaving.

surprised by her reaction, and was unsettled because the expected did not happen! She dominated the conversation by talking about people in the neighborhood, jobs, and other superficial topics. Once outside her building, she thanked the male for walking with her and immediately went into her building (Fig. 5.8).

Later that evening, that same male committed a very violent sexual assault against another female. What was the difference between this woman and the female who became a victim? The woman who avoided the assault was not intimated or overly aggressive. She did the unexpected by humanizing herself, controlling the situation, and manipulating the male to an environment where she could be safe.

The female who became a victim confronted the male as he approached. She yelled at him and asked what he was doing. He answered by slapping her face and calling her a bitch. (Do not ask a question to which the response could be an answer you do not want to hear.) She screamed and attempted to hit the man. He avoided her attempts at defense, beat her face to shut off her screams, and dragged her into a vacant area. The male later left his victim, battered and sodomized.

A Type II assailant cannot allow himself to be physically defeated by a female. This would only reinforce his feelings of inadequacy. The female who was raped provoked aggression, whereas this female defused it and took control of the situation. Once again, if her tactics had failed she could have physically defeated the male with the final 'C'.

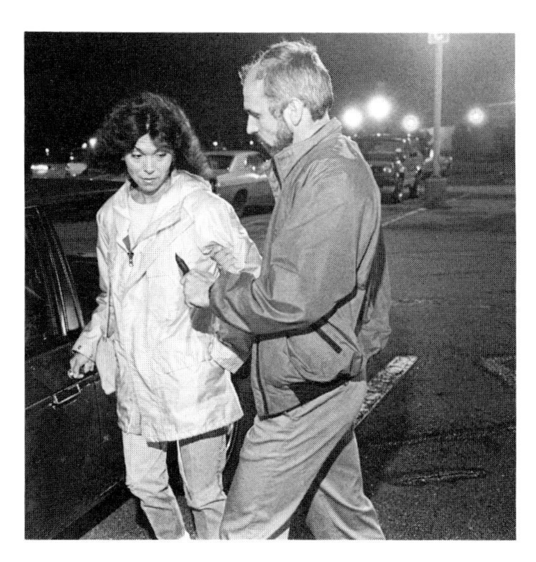

Figure 5.9 ■ Male holding knife—Intimidation.

■ ■ ■ ■

Another example involves a lawyer employed by a firm in Chicago. This woman was walking to her car after meeting with a client one night, when a male approached her in the parking lot and asked directions to a certain building. She told him the way and then began to leave. He grabbed her arm and told her that if she did not go with him, he would kill her. At that point, all she could do was look at the knife he was holding and say nothing (Fig. 5.9). She was afraid, yet found confidence in the fact that she had trained for situations like this and knew what to do. As they were getting into his car she said, "My name is Karen. You don't really believe you need that knife to control me, do you? Come on, put it down. Don't hurt me, I'll do whatever you say! I've had a hell of a day, and now, this!" This did two things: first, it gave her a name and took her from being an object to being human. Secondly, by asking the man if he really needed the knife to control her, she manipulated the male into putting the knife down. Why? If he did not put the knife away, he would have admitted to her and himself that he was afraid of her. This is unacceptable to a male who is trying to dominate and make up for feelings of inadequacy—he will not put himself down by continuing to threaten her with a knife.

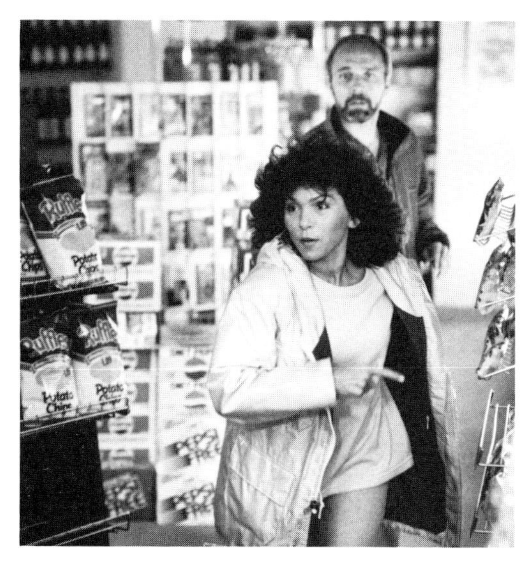

Figure 5.10 ▪ Scene in store with woman escaping.

Once in the car, she started to take control of the situation. She moved the focus from what was happening, to other subjects. She told the male how upset she was with some people, taxes, inflation, etc. She then said she could use a drink to relax. At that point, she stated, "How about stopping at a store for some beer or wine? I'll buy! There's a place just ahead on the left. Pull in." The man was put off balance by her willingness to be with him, and by her giving directions where to turn and stop.

As he was stopping, she reached into her purse and pulled out some money to pay for the beer. They both got out of the car and went into the store. While walking toward the refrigerator, she pulled away and ran around behind the counter (Fig. 5.10), yelling to everyone that she was being kidnapped. Males in the store came to her, while the potential rapist fled. Later, the police arrested the man.

Let's look again at what she did that was so successful. First, she talked to the man and showed herself to be a human being, not an object to be abused. Secondly, she manipulated the man into putting the knife down. And finally, she was in such control of the situation that she was able to get him to stop at a store, allowing her to escape to a place of safety.

■ ■ ■ ■

Another former student was jogging one afternoon when a male ran up beside her. As they approached a secluded area the man started making sexual statements concerning their taking a break in the woods. She had thought about this type of situation quite often and quickly put her rehearsal into practice. She said, "You surprised me. I can't believe this! I've been fantasizing about this happening for weeks! Tell you what—I'm all sweaty and you're no rose yourself. I'll race you back to the 7–11. We can buy some wine and then go to my apartment to shower and enjoy each other." With that she turned and started running to a nearby store. The man couldn't believe her reaction. He let her go and, in fact, started racing her to the store. Once they got there, she jumped behind the counter and started yelling at the potential rapist. He ran out.

She did not react the way the rapist expected which caused him to be off balance and consequently, more easily manipulated.

■ ■ ■ ■

A flight attendant for a major airline was going to her hotel room after a flight. There was a man in the hall close to her room who seemed to be fumbling with his door key. As she opened her door the stranger forced his way in with her. Visibly startled, yet still in control, she said, "Hold it, you must be looking for the party I heard down the hall." The male responded by slapping her and telling her what he wanted. She told him that he didn't need to hurt her to get what he wanted. She then told him she loved aggressive sex, but would like to have something to drink first. Again, this statement defused the aggression and took the man off guard. She followed by asking him to go with her down to the lounge for a drink—all the while moving toward the door. He told her to stop, that he didn't want to go to the bar. She said that was okay with her, she would just as soon order a couple drinks from room service. She moved to the phone, called room service and ordered. When she hung up she told the man that they would be right up. She then began talking about her job and anything else she could think of to buy a few minutes. When the drinks arrived she went to her purse saying she'd buy and then answered the door. As soon as she opened the door, she yelled and ran out. The rapist ran the other way, and the waiter remained, in shock.

Let's look at what she did. This was a part of her job that made her feel vulnerable. She played the "What if . . . ?" game and covered many scenarios. In this specific situation, realizing that she could not convince the man to let her leave the room, the next best thing was to get someone to come to her. She had thought of this ahead of time and was able to pull it off.

■ ■ ■ ■

The final situation involves a woman who was at a small party with some friends and acquaintances. Later in the evening, people began pairing off and eventually this woman was alone with a guy she did not really know. They talked for awhile and within a few minutes he became aggressive and tried to get her to lay on the couch with him. She responded by telling him assertively, that he seemed like a nice guy but that she wasn't interested in laying with him on the couch! The man became more aggressive and pulled her to him. She said, "Hold your horses a minute, I may be interested in playing around with you but this is certainly not the place—they're too many people who could come in on us. Tell you what, let's go get something to eat and then go back to my place." She then got up and grabbed the man's arm to get him to his feet and out the door with her. She told him she lived close by and that they could grab some champagne on the way. While they were walking to the store she controlled the conversation by talking about very superficial things. Once they got to the store she quietly confronted the man with his behavior. She told him she didn't appreciate his attitude and she then told him to leave. He argued for a minute and then left. She then called a friend to come and pick her up.

She was able to control the man until they got to an area where she felt comfortable confronting him.

SUMMARY

The effectiveness of these 'C's' cannot be overstated. They are designed to counter steps in the rape sequence that rapists follow.

The male targets a female who appears vulnerable to him, and attempts to dominate her—expecting Fight or Fright. By using these 'C's', you are defusing the aggression, taking control, and manipulating the entire situation so that it is transformed from a male controlled scenario to a scene controlled *by you.*

Remember, they are only as good as you are! Look at your lifestyle and practice the "What If . . . ?" game in those situations where you may be vulnerable. Don't kid yourself into thinking that you can come up with some clever statements utilizing the principles without ever practicing. *You must practice* these principles and mentally rehearse in order to use them to their greatest potential.

If they succeed, you are unhurt and free of the male. If they are not succeeding, you are buying time while maneuvering into a position from which to physically defeat him. I have had many former students contact me concerning assault attempts aimed at them. Eighty-five percent were able to eliminate the conflict through the use of these principles, and 15% had to rely on the final 'C.' All prevented themselves from being victimized.

If you fight first, there are no other options available to you should you lose!! A fact, unfortunately, that many victims of rape have discovered too late.

Chapter 5 Worksheet

When are the times in your life when you feel the most vulnerable? Playing the "What if . . . ?" game, describe in detail what you would do if. . . . Be specific—do not just say that you would be confident and take control. How would you control? What would you say?

CHAPTER

6

TRANSITION—THE BRIDGE BETWEEN TALK AND FIGHT

I had always been kind of hard line when it came to the "Four C's" and rapists. I felt that no matter what the situation, if your attempts to defeat the man psychologically with Confidence and Control failed or you were not given a chance to use them, you should immediately move into the final 'C'—Complete Incapacitation. You don't ask to be a victim, so why be concerned about him!!

I soon learned that there is a need for something to say/do when Confidence and Control are not working and you feel it is not yet appropriate to move into the fourth 'C'. More times than not, this involves situations in which the man is known to the woman. Call him a date, acquaintance or whatever label you want to use—she is generally going to feel the need to exhaust all possible resources before choosing to use Complete Incapacitation. Thus, the birth of *Transition*.

There are many variables associated with Transition. Each situation involves different personalities and calls for you to figure out

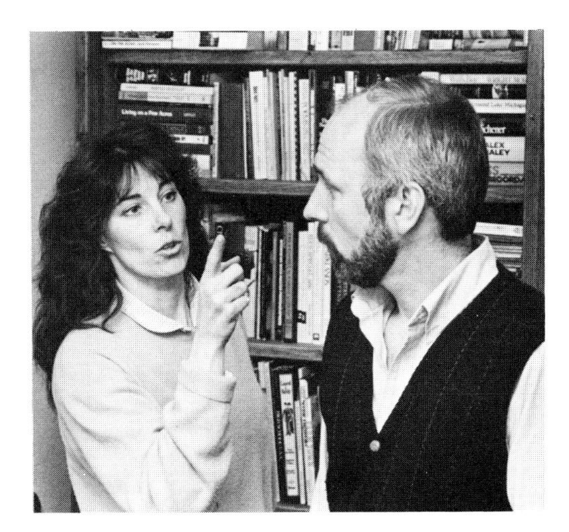

Figure 6.1 ▪ Male intimidated and backing down.

if Transition is applicable, if you want to use it, and specifically, how to apply it.

Transition involves three courses of action that you can take. The first is to try to reason with the man, attempting to make him feel guilty. The feeling of guilt *may* override his need for power and sexual gratification. Reasoning can be attempted whether the man is a stranger or familiar to you. Realistically, however, the better known the man is to you, the greater the effectiveness of attempts at reasoning with him. By saying something like, "Come on, Bill, think how you will feel tomorrow. You're not the kind of guy who needs to force someone into sex are you? I know you're not, and so do you. I'm going to leave now and forget this ever happened." By doing this, you defuse aggression and change the focus from his gratification, to more humanistic feelings, enabling you to move away from him.

Two other actions you can use in Transition involve aggression. Aggression can be either verbal, physical, or both. Whichever form you use, use it with caution because aggression asks for a response from the male. He will either be intimidated by it and back down, possibly negotiating (Fig. 6.1), or he may decide to fight it (Fig. 6.2).

Because each situation is different, you must sense what may or may not work. Predicting how anyone would react when confronted

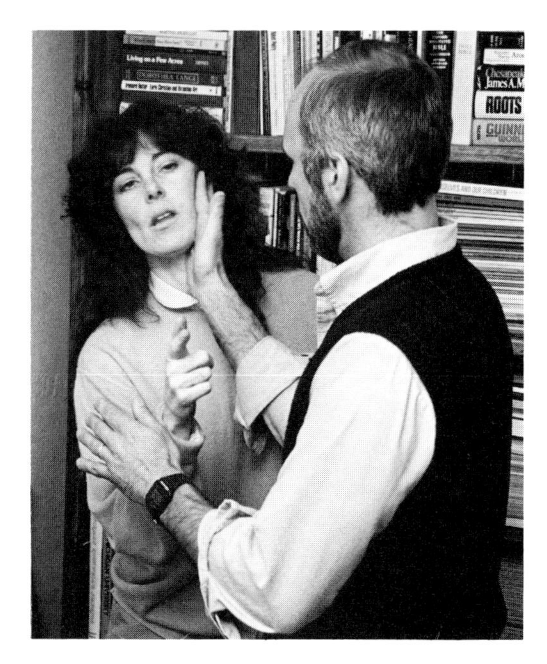

Figure 6.2 ▪ Male responding aggressively.

with aggression is difficult, but even more so the less you know the person.

Verbal techniques should center on making it clear to the man that you do not appreciate his behavior, you are not going to allow it to continue, and you are going to leave, or demand that he leaves, whichever the case.

Physically aggressive techniques can take many forms. If you want to use martial arts, weapons, street fighting tactics, etc., NOW would be the time to use them. Be realistic about your skills! Once you are physical, the situation turns dynamic—bodies are in motion. Dealing with someone who is generally bigger, stronger, and more street experienced is not easy.

Regardless of your choice of aggressive techniques *always* follow them up with attempting to get away from the situation. Do not, for example, yell and push at the man while remaining on the couch—move to the door!! By moving away from him, you lessen his control over you and the situation

■ ■ ■ ■

Now let's look at some examples of how Transition is put into practice.

A 20 year old student of mine was in a situation involving a man with whom she had once gone out. They both lived in a college residence hall and one night he was visiting her room. Her roommates were gone and would not be back for hours. The two of them talked for a while and then began to kiss. It wasn't long before he attempted to become sexually intimate. She told him that she was not interested at this time, and asked him not to ruin what they had. He became more aggressive telling her that she was a tease and that she really wanted him. Showing a side of himself that she had not seen before, she became concerned and moved into Control. She said, "Slow down, I don't know what you have in mind exactly but there's plenty of time. Tell you what, maybe I was a bit hasty. I need to be more relaxed. Let's go to the store and get a bottle of champagne." She made a move to get up. He stopped her and said he wanted to have sex now. She attempted to regain control, but was having no success. This woman then moved into Transition by saying, "Stop it! I don't want to do this with you. Sometime, maybe, but not now! You don't need to force a person in order to get sex, do you? Leave, now!!"While she was saying all this, she was moving away from the man. Once she got some space between them she jumped up and went to the door. She opened it and once again, yelled at him to leave. He got up, protested, and left.

This woman used two aspects of Transition in order to get away from him. She was aggressive in her statements and yet, was reasoning with him by appealing to his ego saying that he didn't need to use force to get sex. It worked very well for her.

■ ■ ■ ■

Another female, was out with her date and another couple. Later in the evening the four of them went back to her date's apartment to play cards. The other couple soon left. This woman and her date started engaging in sexual intimacies. A point was reached at which

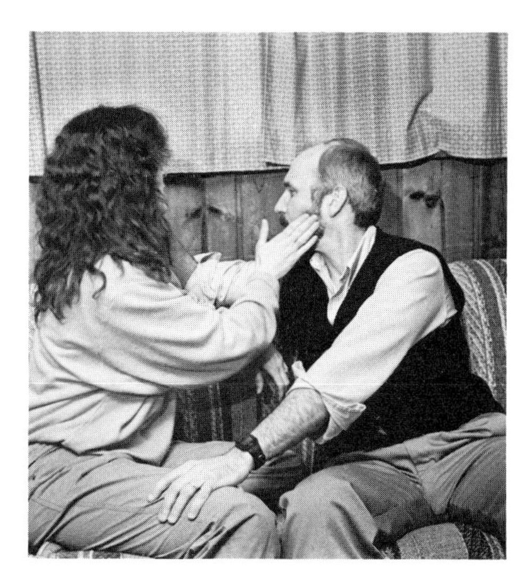

Figure 6.3 ■ Female yelling and confronting male.

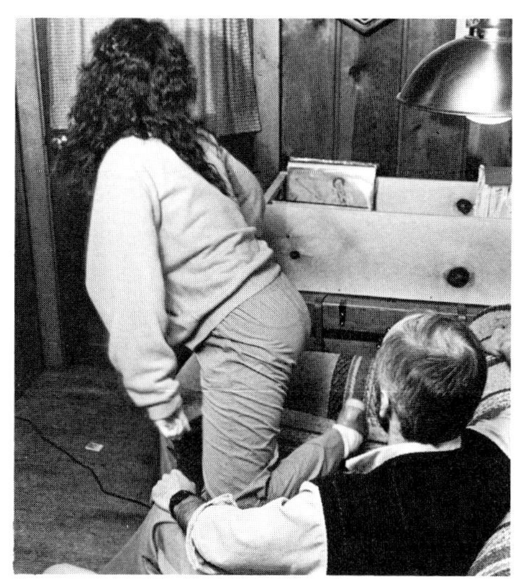

Figure 6.4 ■ Female leaving the situation.

she wanted to stop. He ignored her and tried to get her to submit to him. She moved into control and tried to talk him into going for some champagne. He refused and continued with his attempts to get her to have sex with him. She became angry and yelled for him to stop while at the same time, pushing him away. She then slapped him and confronted him with behaving like a selfish animal. (Fig. 6.3) She followed this by getting off the couch and leaving. (Fig. 6.4)

This woman had tried everything possible to get around people so that she could talk with him about his behavior, but he refused which forced her into Transition. Fortunately, her aggression did not cause him to become violent.

SUMMARY

The basic idea of Transition is to attempt to reason with the man by playing on guilt, and/or to use some form of verbal or physical aggression designed to stop his behavior and allow you to move away from him. Transition is both realistic and applicable and the success rate improves in proportion to how well known the man is to you. I have found it rare for a man, whom the intended victim knows well, to continue once she moves into Control or into Transition.

As in Confidence and Control, your success depends upon your believability and ability to regain control over the situation. It is important for you to mentally practice situations where you see yourself using Transition—What do you say? How do you say it? And, what do you do? Practice!!

Remember, this phase of the Four 'C's' gives you and the man a final chance to break the assault sequence before you are forced into the decision to use your "trump card"—the fourth 'C'—Complete Incapacitation.

CHAPTER

7

COMPLETE INCAPACITATION—YOUR FOURTH AND FINAL 'C'

If Control has been used without success, or the male is not giving you time to use the psychological principles of Control (i.e., he is choking you, hitting, etc.), the only way to get out of the rape sequence is to fight back and to do so effectively, not randomly.

Before getting into the techniques of this option, it is important to understand several factors relating specifically to physical resistance in sexual assault.

ATTACK AREA MISCONCEPTIONS

The first factor that must be considered is to clear up misconceptions about parts of the male anatomy to attack. From an offensive standpoint, there are only two areas on the male body that can be attacked which will incapacitate a Type II rapist (Violent Sexual Attack). Almost anything you do will defeat a Type I rapist (Sexual Confrontation), but a Type II must be completely incapacitated to be defeated. In my opinion, the reason so much emphasis is put on knee kicking, nose striking, foot stomping, and many other methods of resistance, is that they were and are done successfully with Type I assailants. If you were to look at the most recent statistics, the best that can be said is that a female has about a 60 percent chance of getting away if she uses these types of confrontational techniques. Unfortunately, the statistics do not give a representation of how many of the women in that 60 percent were hurt even though they got away. Or, of what happened to the 40 percent who did not get away. Fifty-fifty or sixty-forty are not statistics that can be lived with—I cannot accept or condone a system which says that if 100 women were to physically confront a rapist, approximately 40 would completely fail and some of the remaining 60 would be hurt.

To be successful, you must attack areas of the body which will incapacitate, not just inflict pain. Almost every book on rape prevention has a picture like this (Fig. 7.1), showing the countless areas on a male body that can be attacked

This picture makes us believe that the male body is very vulnerable when, in fact, **IN AN ASSAULT, IT IS NOT!!** Not only is it extremely difficult to hit any of these areas, but remember the male has enkeflin, adrenalin, and pain gates within his body, all of which are geared toward suppressing or temporarily masking his pain. You cannot just inflict pain, you must incapacitate!!

Let's look at some of the more common areas of the body you are told to attack.

Nose. One of the most overrated attack areas. Women are told to hit up into the nose driving a piece of bone into the brain or at least causing sufficient pain to make him leave you alone. Bull!! I have seen

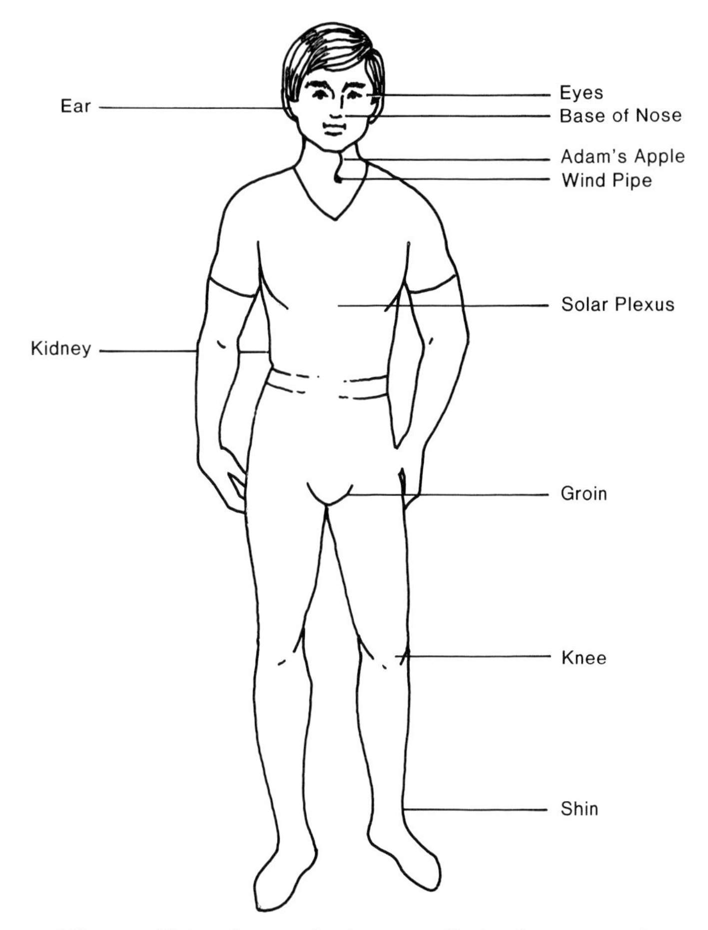

Figure 7.1 ■ Areas to incapacitate the sexual assailant.

males in fights in which their nose was broken so that it practically came out of their ear, yet it did not stop them. It causes pain and the eyes to water, but generally will not incapacitate.

Ears. The idea of attacking this area is that you cup the hand and strike both ears simultaneously. The theory is that it will rupture the tympanic membrane (ear drum), causing extreme pain and extreme dizziness. This again is a fallacy—ask any scuba diver. The tympanic membrane can rupture and a person barely feels it for a period of time. Eventual pain possibly, incapacitation—no.

Throat. Although the throat would appear to be very vulnerable, in a stress situation, it is not. I have studied fights in which the ages of the males range from 4 years to 23 years old. The males dropped their chins and thus eliminated the throat as a vulnerable area. This is done instinctively, without thought. Plus, most victims are shorter than the rapist, which causes him to look down thus, covering the throat area automatically.

Solar Plexus. A moving target is the size of a 50 cent piece. A very, very low success area for being struck effectively. If you miss what do you say, "Boy, what well toned chest muscles."? You do not get many second chances.

Floating Rib. Where is it? What is it?

Kidneys. Seldom does a male attack someone with his back to them. The force needed to hurt someone by hitting the kidney area is tremendous.

Knee. Probably the most single overrated area. Unless the male attacks with locked knees (Fig. 7.2), they simply are not vulnerable.

I have done many demonstrations where females have kicked my knees as hard as they could—no success. I have even had a female black belt attempt to harm my knees as though in a typical assault situation, again, to no avail. In fighting situations, the knees are bent. The force necessary to damage them enough to incapacitate, is beyond the capabilities of all but the most skilled black belt.

Ankles, Toes, and Hands. Distracting and pain inducing but definitely not incapacitating to a Type II.

Groin. One of the two best areas if you know how to attack it correctly. Many nerve endings, and despite the disagreement of many males—no muscle. When attacked effectively, it overrides enkeflin, adrenaline, drugs, and anger. The author believes that there is only one, 100 percent effective, way to attack the groin

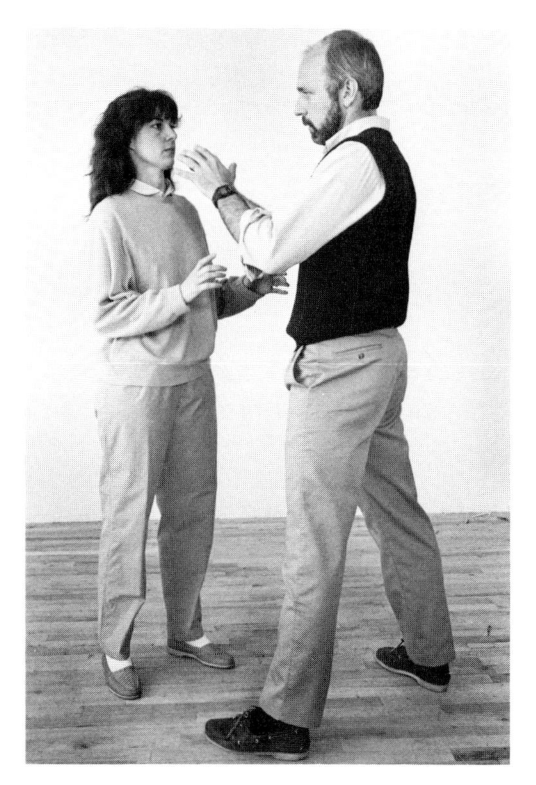

Figure 7.2 ■ Male standing with locked knees.

(you will be told of it later). Suffice it to say, kicking and striking are very low success techniques unless you are highly trained. This is an area that the male expects will be kicked at so, he is wary. Also, by kicking at the groin area, you place yourself in an extremely unbalanced and, therefore, more vulnerable position.

Eyes. The single best area to attack, if done properly, will be given to you later. High concentration of nerve endings, and no muscle. Effective attack will override drugs, etc. Unfortunately, most females do not know the proper way to attack. They generally end up further enraging the male.

When attacking the male body, it is essential that you use the highest success techniques against the most vulnerable areas of the body. Complete incapacitation is the surest way to prevent yourself from being harmed. Techniques that do not achieve this end, are potentially very dangerous to the women using them. This is due to the fact that if, and when, they do not work, the male becomes further enraged and alerted to the fact that you are going to try to harm him.

■ ■ ■ ■

Now that we have deleted the areas of the body which it is fairly useless to attack, and techniques of attacking those areas which do not work, let's get to the heart of this option. The use of your body as a weapon—Complete Incapacitation.

These techniques are *extremely* simple and designed for close in, completely incapacitating defense. There is no such thing as fighting to drive the man away—with this attitude, you run a high chance of failure. If you decide to use your body as a weapon, it must be with the intent to win.

The two techniques you will be given have been in use for hundreds of years. To my knowledge, they have never failed when used.

The techniques are, Thumbs to Eyes and Testicle Crush. Sounds pretty bad doesn't it? Do you think a rapist gives a damn about the effect the assault will have on the female? If a male chooses to attempt to mentally and physically use and abuse a female, he must suffer the consequences for his actions. Remember, if you have to use these techniques, you are most probably dealing with a Violent Sexual Attack (Type II). Your success is determined by your desire to win.

This 'C' should give you confidence, for if used, it will be completely effective. Unless the man has glass eyes or no testicles, I've never heard of a rape situation in which the eyes or groin were not exposed for attack. They are always going to be close by—somewhere!! (Fig. 7.3.)

Once the hand or hands are in position to either crush a testicle or drive the thumbs into the eyes, there is no way your success can be prevented. Unless you are being hurt, do not fight (other than psychologically as described in Control, until the eyes or groin can be attacked. The man should not be aware that you are going to attack.

It may be necessary to manipulate the man into believing that you are willing to kiss and/or touch him. As disgusting as this may be, it's better than being raped. You may have to make certain compromises in

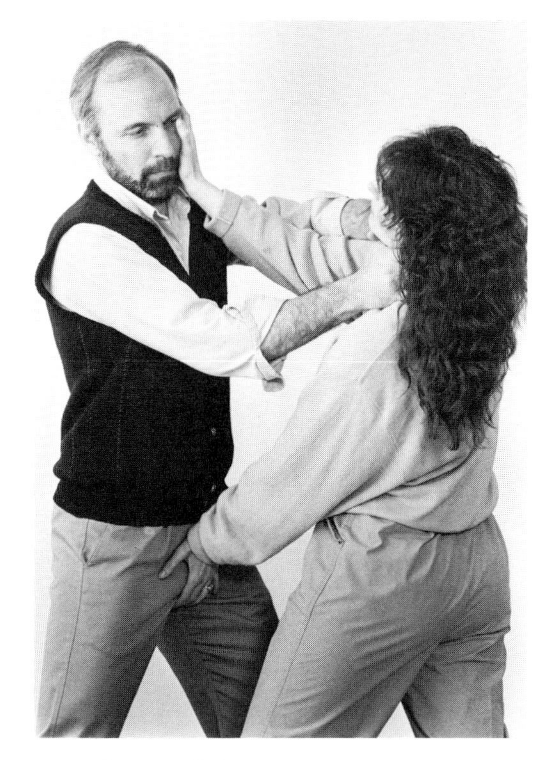

Figure 7.3. ■ Picture of man covering up.

order to come out a winner. Approximately 70 percent of all sexual assaults involve oral sex—what better chance—it is a perfect opportunity to crush a testicle having convinced the man you are willing to comply.

Though the technique may seem easy, there are a few things you must learn in order to insure their success.

THUMBS TO EYES

Remember, if the psychological techniques and transition are not working, or you are not given time to use them, your goal for this technique is to bring the tips of your fingers to the jaw line of the male. (Figs 7.4, 7.5, 7.6.)

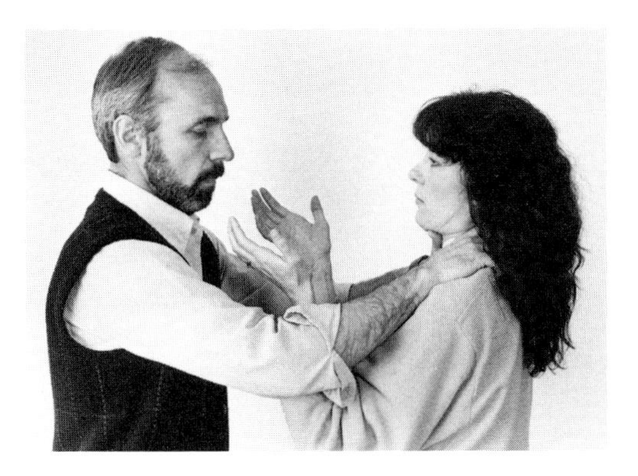

Figure 7.4.

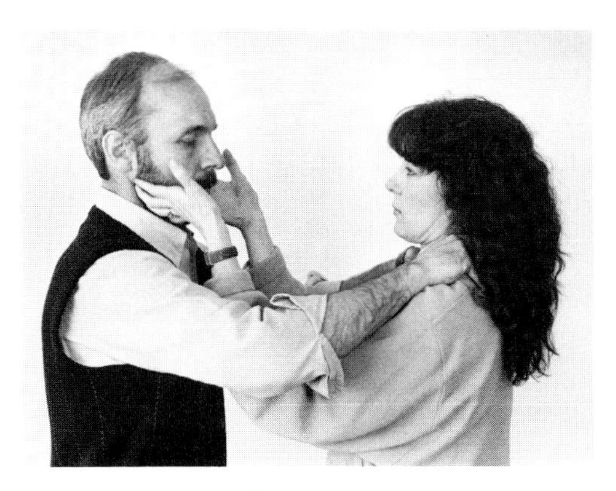

Figure 7.5.

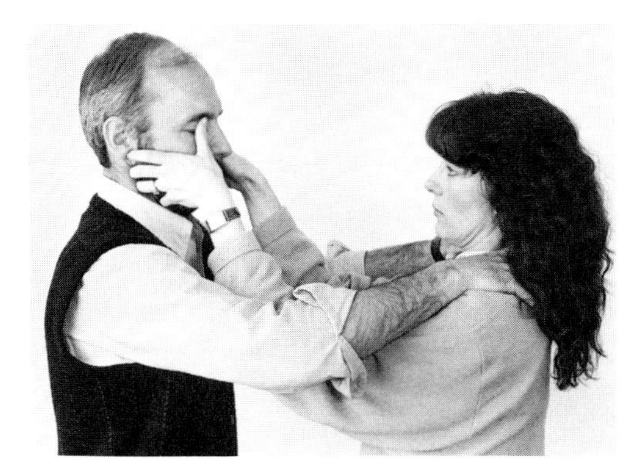

Figure 7.6.

Figure 7.4, 7.5, and 7.6 ■ Sequence showing technique.

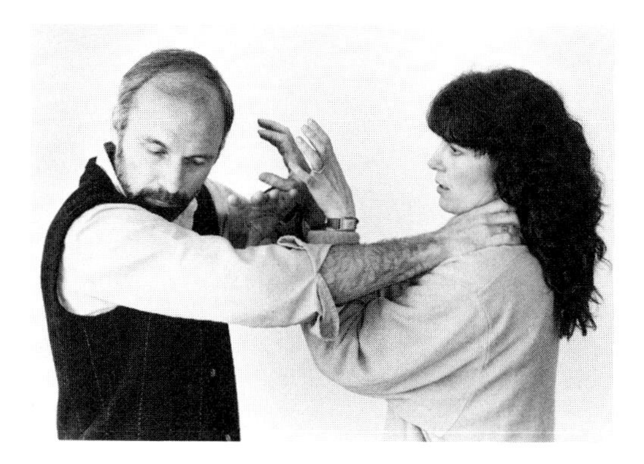

Figure 7.7 ■ Picture of going straight for the eyes—Wrong.

By doing this, you have not alerted the male to the fact that you are going to attack the eyes. If you go straight for the eyes, (Fig. 7.7) the male could respond by turning his head or blocking your arms. It is threatening to see fingers or thumbs coming toward the eyes, but bringing the hands under the chin to the upper jaw area is non-threatening (Fig. 7.8).

Once your hands are in position, drive the thumbs around and into the eye socket. The all or none principle is imperative—either do it as fast as you can and drive the thumb as deep as you can, or do not do it. Do not be concerned as to where in the socket, or what part of the thumb to use. Simply drive the thumbs around and in!

The technique takes less than a second and is 100 percent effective. It has never failed to completely incapacitate. Once done, the male will drop to the ground and go into shock—immediately. There is virtually no chance that he will be able to harm you. In fact, he will need medical assistance.

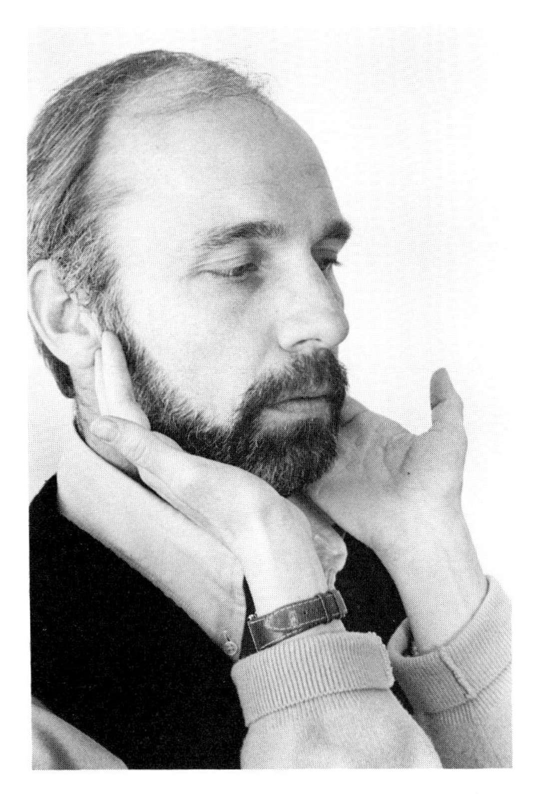

Figure 7.8 ■ Enlargement of hands under chin to jaw—Correct.

TESTICLE CRUSH

With the male wearing pants, it is somewhat difficult to isolate a testicle to crush. Because of this, the eyes, generally, receive first priority for attack unless the testicles are already exposed or unless you can convince the male to expose them.

To succeed with this technique, you simply hold the testicle in the palm of your hand and squeeze as fast and as hard as you can. Again, the all or none principle applies (Figs. 7.9 and 7.10.)

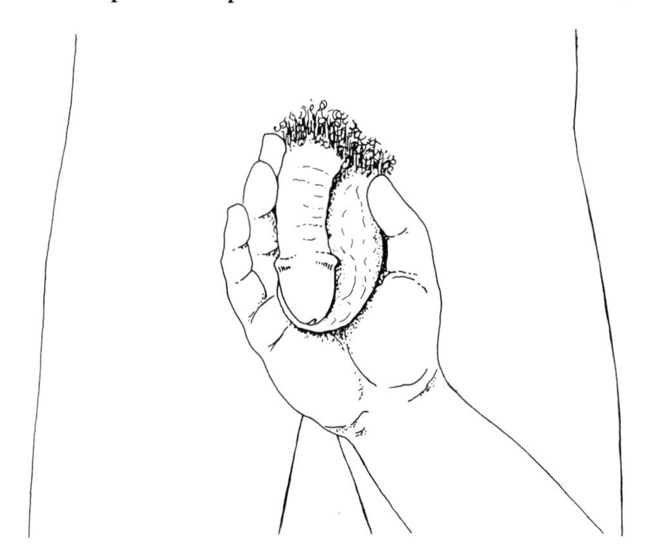

Figure 7.9 ■ Drawing of hand.

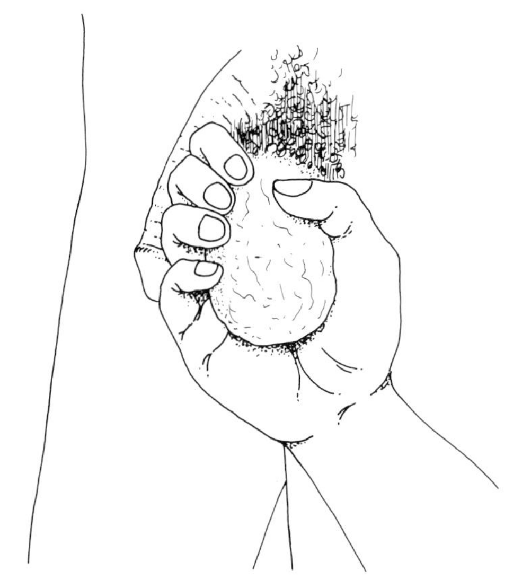

Figure 7.10 ■ Drawing of squeeze.

The hand comes from under the testicle—not in front of it. (Figs. 7.11 and 7.12.)

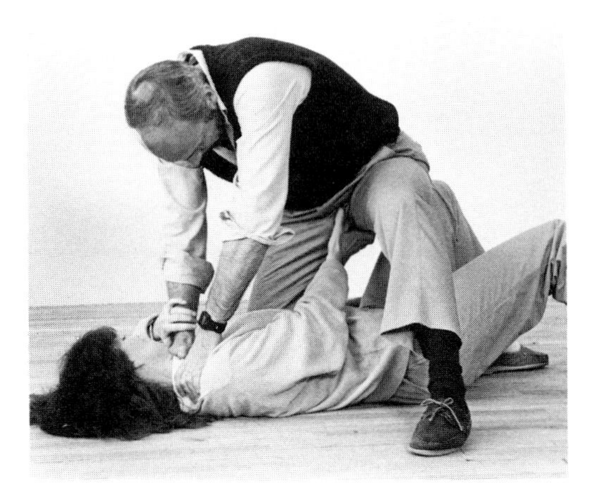

Figure 7.11 ■ Under.

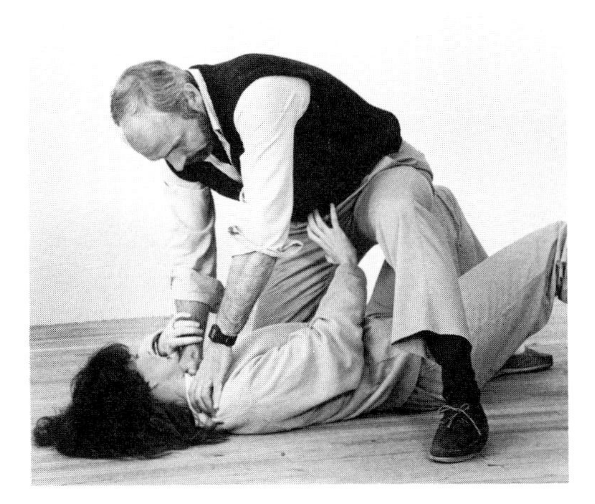

Figure 7.12 ■ In front.

I understand the fear or anxiety the thought of doing either of these techniques creates. You fear they may fail or you feel you could not harm someone in this way. First, a 5 year old child has the strength and speed to do the techniques, so have no doubt about the possibility of success if you decide to use Complete Incapacitation. Secondly, you

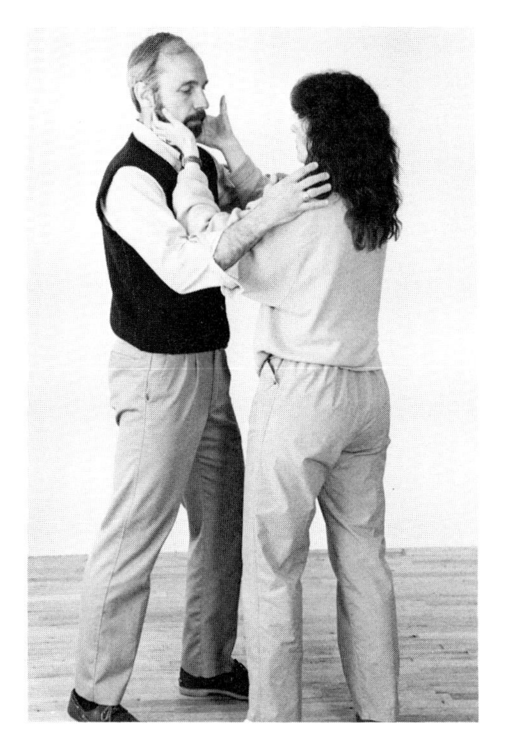

Figure 7.13 ■ Standing.

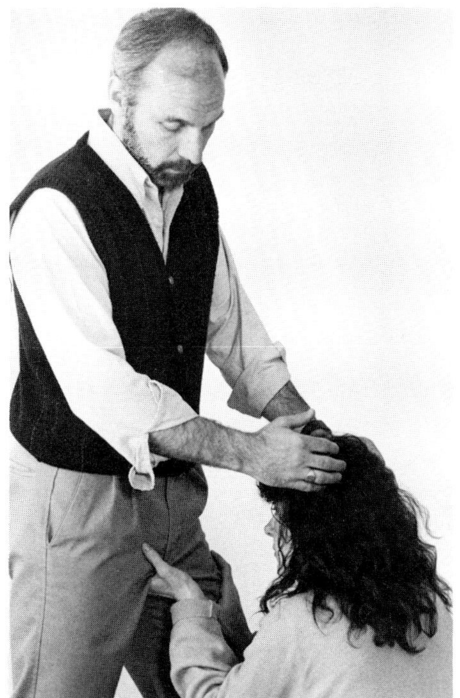

Figure 7.14 ■ Kneeling.

do not ask to be assaulted—ever. The *only* way you can be sure that you will not be among the tens of thousands of victims each year, is with these techniques. No other techniques can give you 100 percent success. It is sad, that women are often concerned about really hurting the male and the male could not care less about the pain and turmoil he causes. Think about yourself and your survival first!!

The goal, in *any* situation where the psychological principles have failed or cannot be used, and the use of your body as a weapon becomes appropriate, is to get one or both hands in contact with one of the two incapacitating areas. It does not matter if you are standing, kneeling, or on the ground. (Figs. 7.13, 7.14, 7.15).

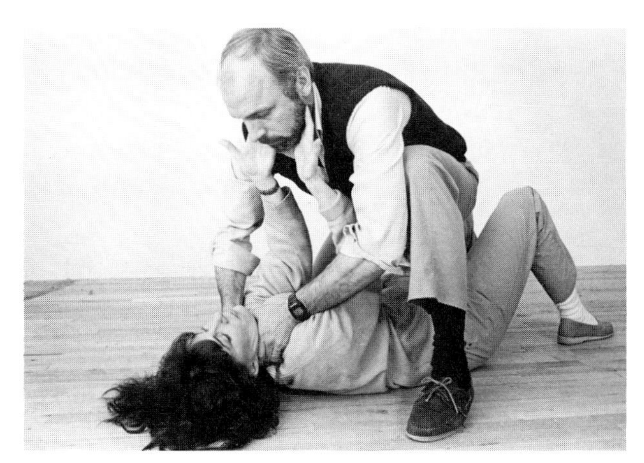

Figure 7.15 ■ On the ground.

No complicated techniques to remember. No confusion as to which technique to use. No chance for failure! He has testicles and eyes, and you have your hands!

Now that you know the techniques which will completely incapacitate, there are a few tactics which you must know to survive a life threatening situation. Survival consists of neutralizing the technique the male is using and then completely incapacitating him.

SURVIVAL

Life threatening situations consist primarily of strangulations or the presence of a weapon. In dealing with these, you have one objective only: to neutralize whatever he is doing to you by completely incapacitating him.

Strangulations

The most important thing to remember if being choked is, *attack!* Sounds difficult, but it really is not. Most people, when choked, try to pry off whatever is choking them. (Figs. 7.16 and 7.17.)

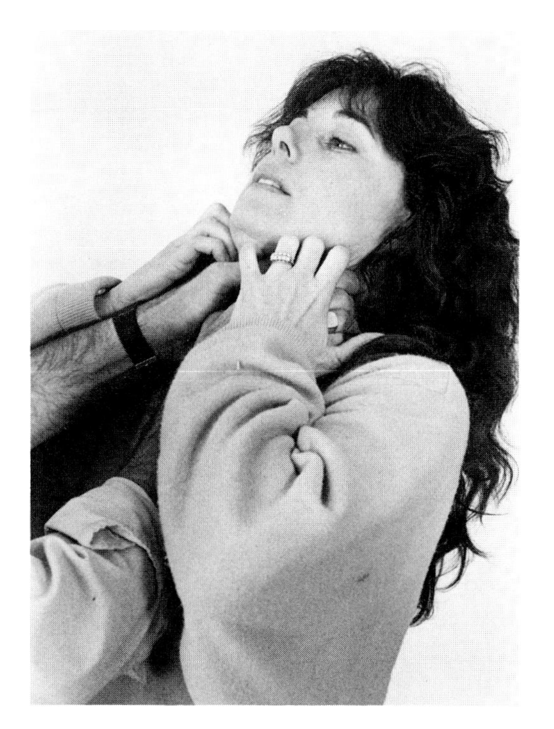

Figure 7.16 ■ Woman grabbing for man's hands.

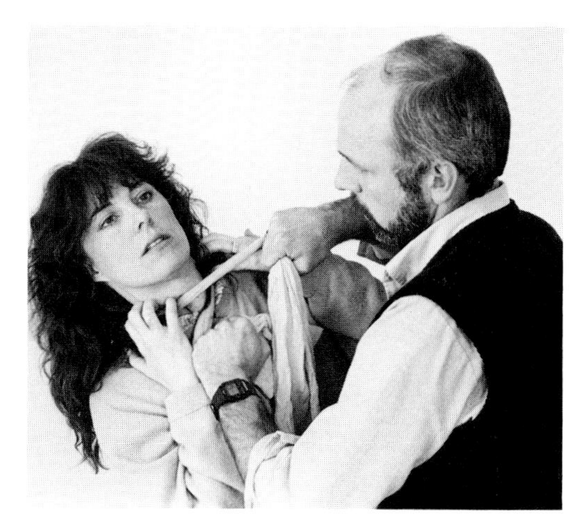

Figure 7.17 ■ Grabbing for garrote.

This uses up vital seconds that you cannot afford to lose. When choked, you will first experience shock and disbelief, then you will experience pain and panic because you will be unable to breathe, then dizziness occurs, and eventually, you will black out. With a strong choke, this whole process will take between four and five seconds. By attempting to pry off what is choking you, you tend to fixate on that and do nothing else until you pass out.

Think about it—if the man's hands are on your throat, they cannot be protecting his vital areas. If you condition yourself to *attack* the choker instead of *attempting defense,* you will win because of his vulnerability.

Front Choke Response

In front chokes, I have found that the man bends his arms to exert maximum force. He is aggressive and because of this his arms are bent. This will put his face within reach of your hands. (Fig. 7.18.)

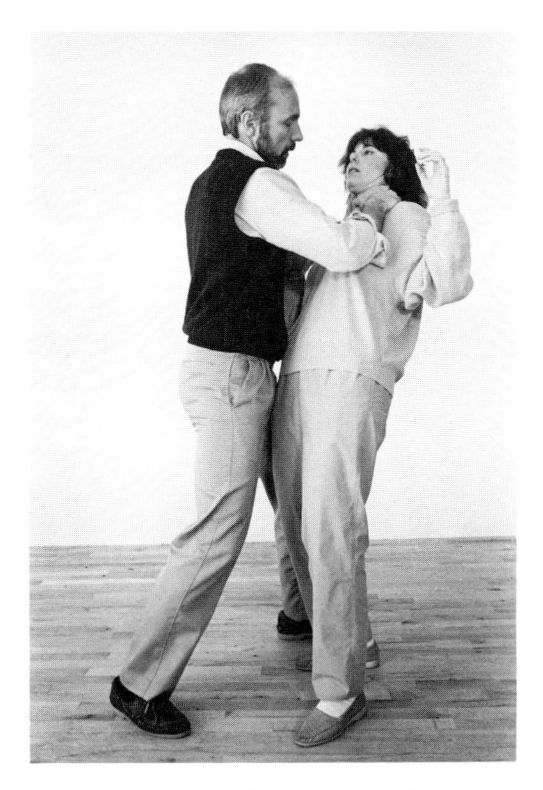

Figure 7.18 ■ Initial grab.

If you can, step back to absorb the force of the male and to gain control. Notice her hands are coming up (Fig. 7.19) reaching for the jaw. She then drives the thumbs around and into the eye sockets. (Fig. 7.20). This whole process takes less than two seconds and will be 100 percent effective.

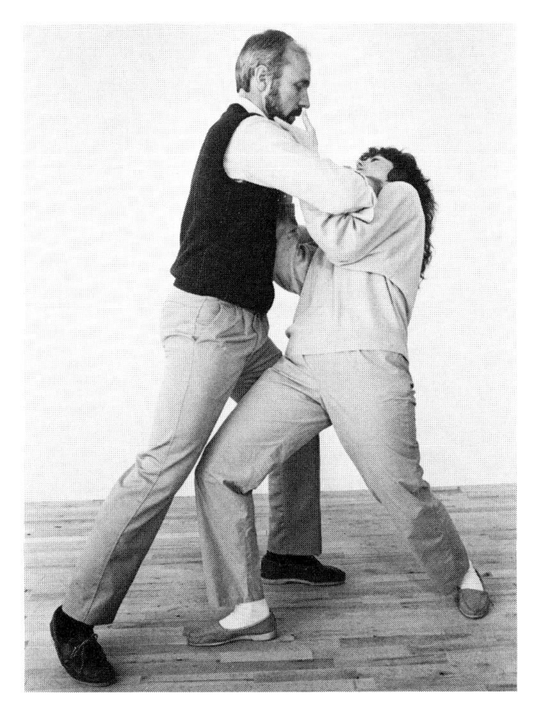

Figure 7.19 ■ Hands coming up.

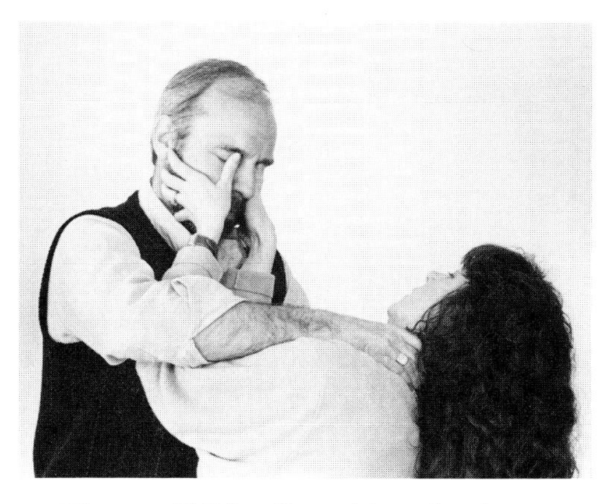

Figure 7.20 ■ Reaching for jaw.

If the male uses a garrote to choke with, the response is the same. The only difference will be that you will be pulled toward him. This is good because, the closer you are, the easier it is to reach the jaw and eyes. Also, you will not be in an off-balance state. (Figs. 7.21, 7.22, 7.23.)

It has been my experience, that most of the time females are choked in a face to face position to the assailant. He wants to see the effect he's having—your fear and pain. This gives him something called psychosexual gratification. Remember—attack, attack, attack!! The male is not expecting a purposeful, direct attack, and he is not defending against it.

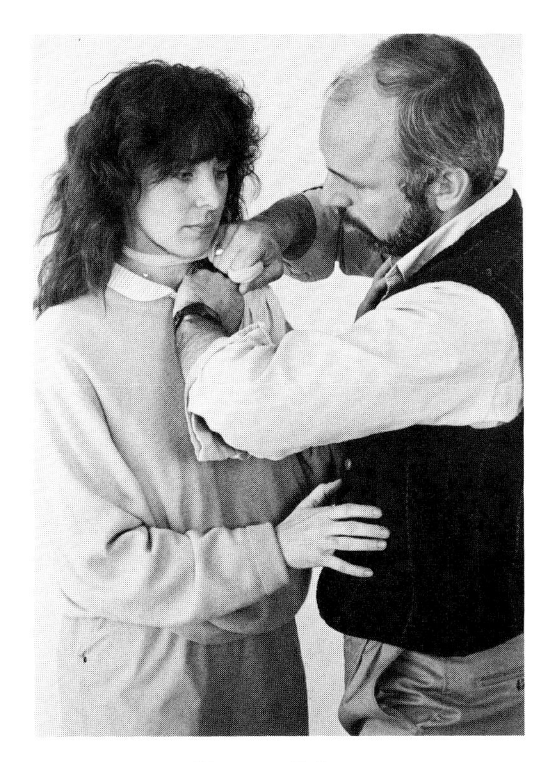

Figure 7.21.

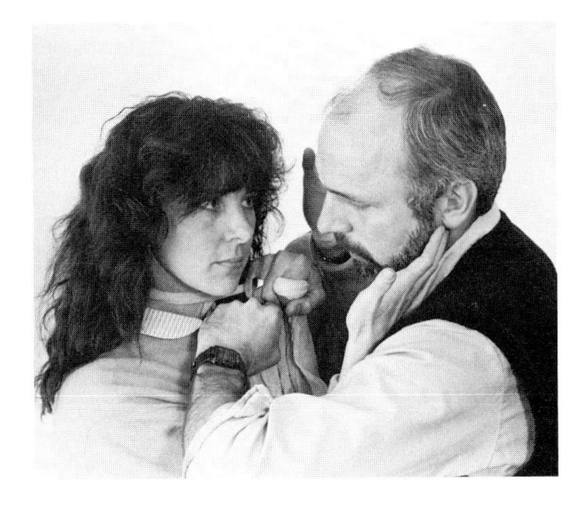

Figure 7.22.

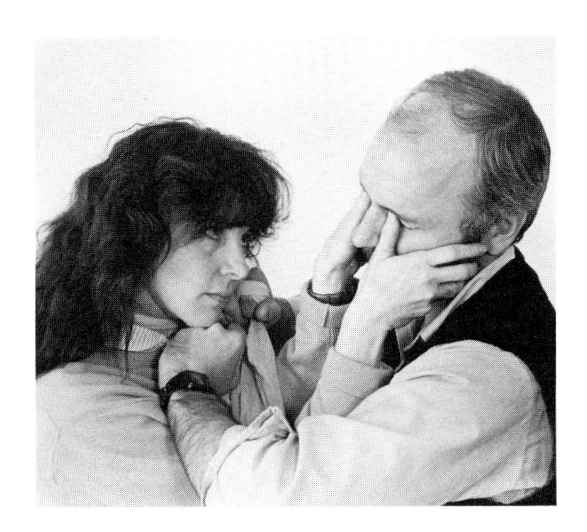

Figure 7.23.

Figures 7.21, 7.22, and 7.23 ■ Sequence showing technique.

If, for whatever reason, you cannot reach the man's jawline, fall to the ground (Figs. 7.24, 7.25, 7.26.) You may already be there!

This will bring the male within reach of your attack. If you cannot reach the eyes, you will be able to reach the testicles. One or the other will be within reach!

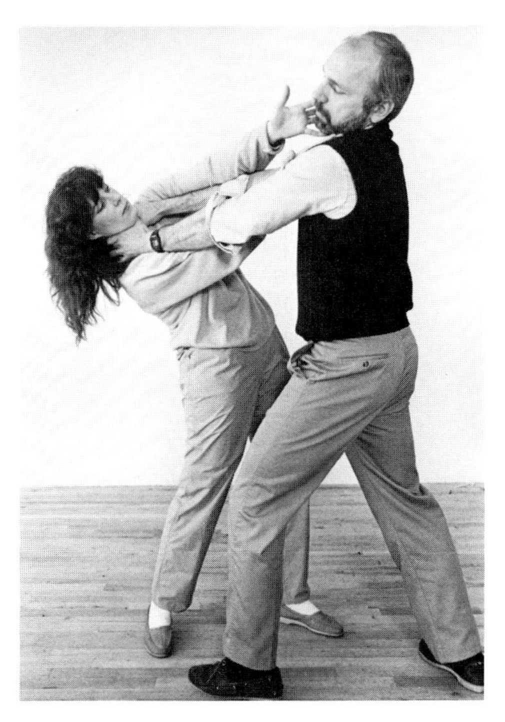

Figure 7.24 ▪ Woman unable to reach.

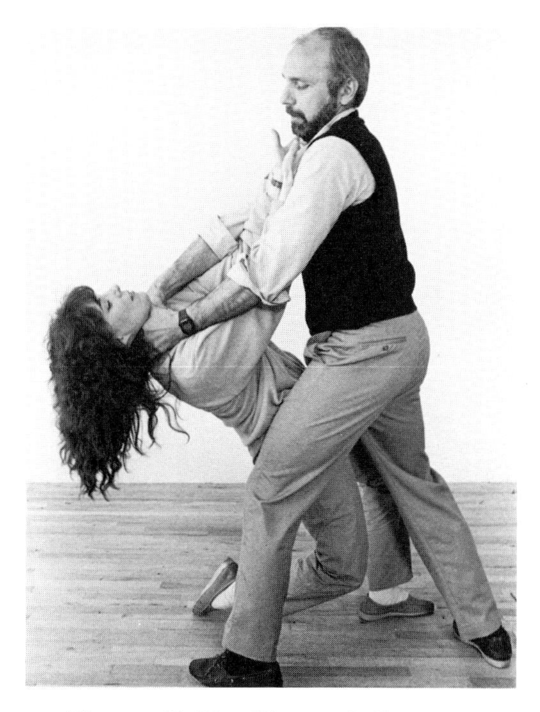

Figure 7.25 ■ Shows falling to ground.

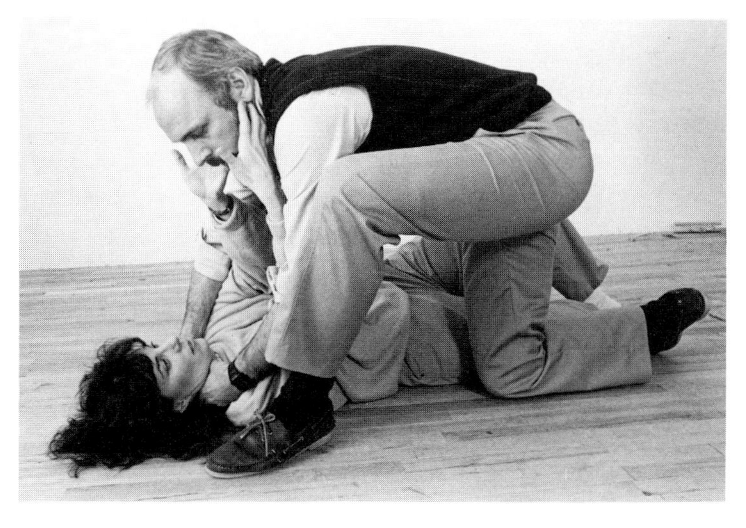

Figure 7.26 ■ On ground, on back, hands on jaws and thumbs poised.

Rear Choke Responses

A choke from the rear is obviously more critical, because you cannot see the attacker. The principle is still the same—do not attempt defense—*attack!* In rear chokes, the face of the male will be very close to your head. It has to be in order for him to exert a force.

Rear Choke with Fingers

In order to choke from behind, using just his hands, the male will be pulling you toward him. Do not attempt defense and grab for his hands—you have plenty of time to win, if you do not panic. (Fig. 7.27.)

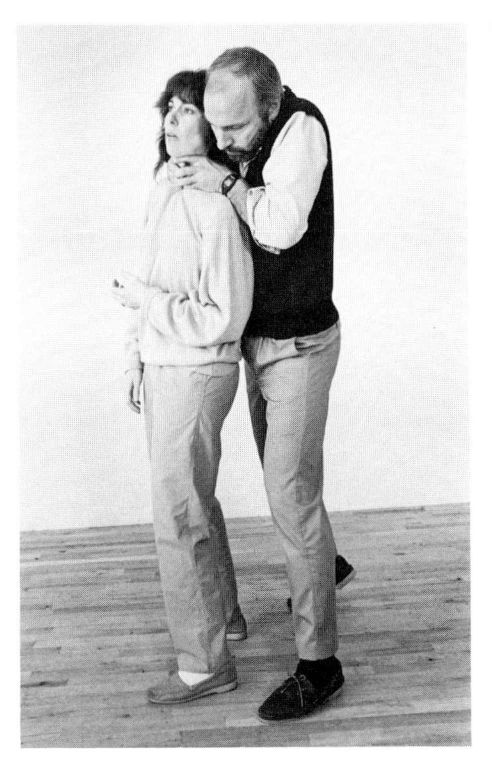

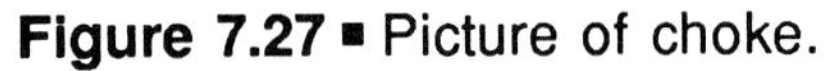

Figure 7.27 ■ Picture of choke.

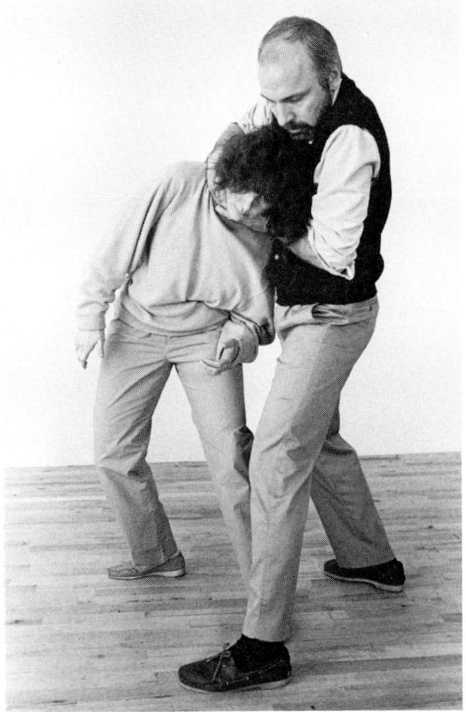

Figure 7.28 ■ Bend and step toward.

When you feel the choke, immediately bend as far to the side as you can while stepping toward the man (Fig. 7.28.) Straighten your body up and face the man. (Fig. 7.29.) This must be done very rapidly. Once you are facing the male, bring your hand or hands to his jaw and drive the thumbs into the eye sockets. (Fig. 7.30.)

If, for whatever reason, you cannot turn to face the male, reach for his testicles. If he has tight pants on, you will probably not be able to completely incapacitate him. However, you may cause him to loosen the choke which would allow you to turn. (Figs. 7.31 and 7.32.)

If the testicles cannot be reached, attempt to make some kind of contact with his eyes. As a last resort, fall to the ground and *roll to your back* in order to be facing him. Then, go for the eyes or testicles. (Figs. 7.33, 7.34, 7.35.)

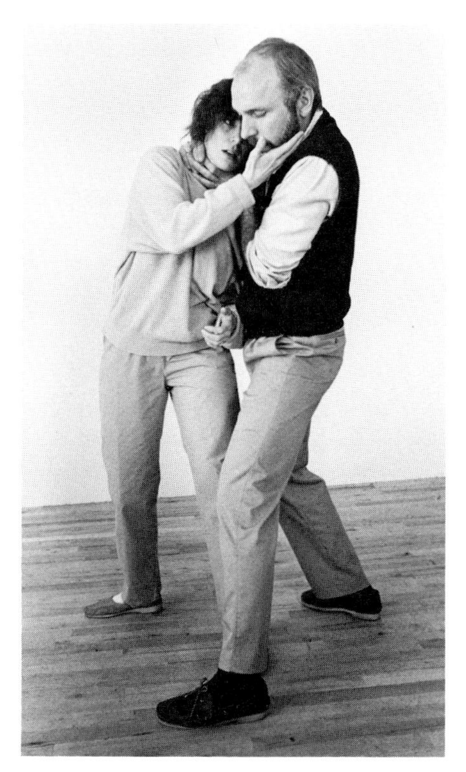

Figure 7.29 ■ Straighten and face.

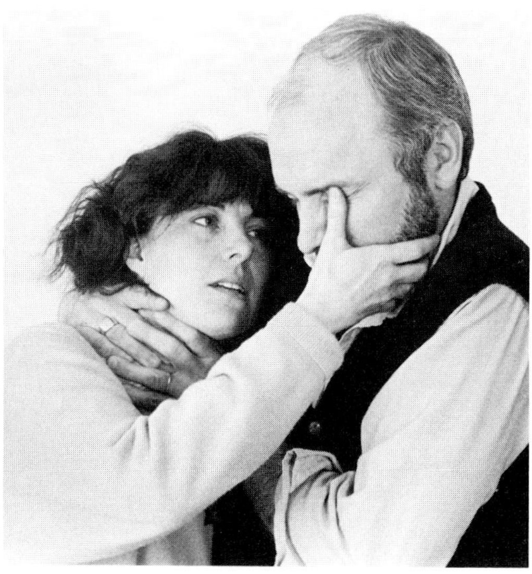

Figure 7.30 ■ Hands to jaw.

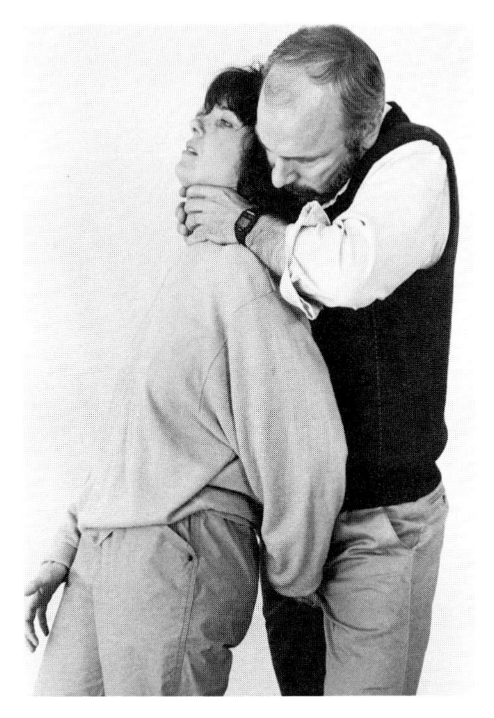

Figure 7.31 ■ Picture of reaching for groin.

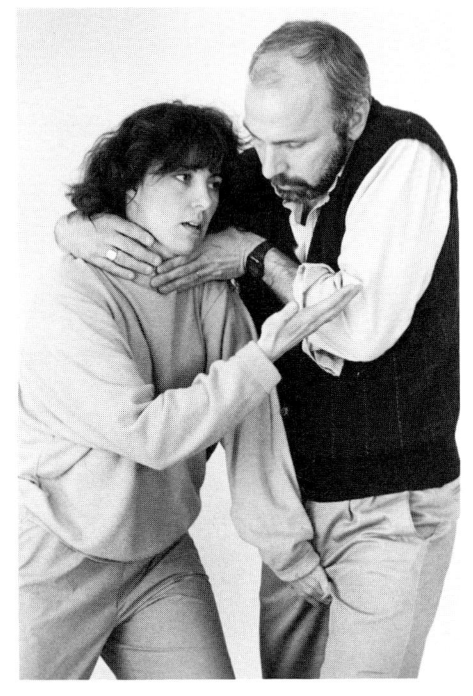

Figure 7.32 ■ Reaching for eyes.

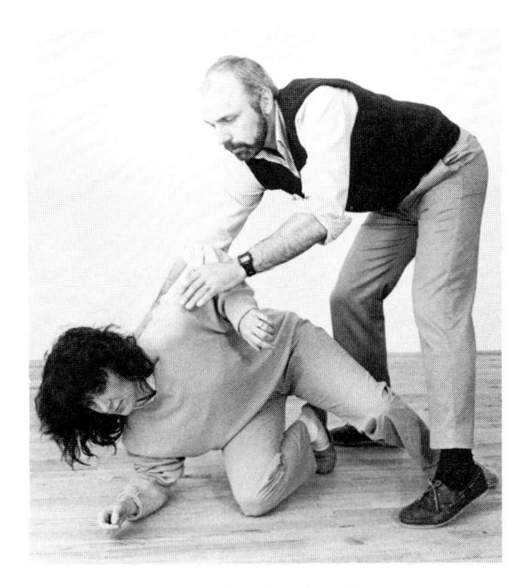

Figure 7.33 ■ Falling.

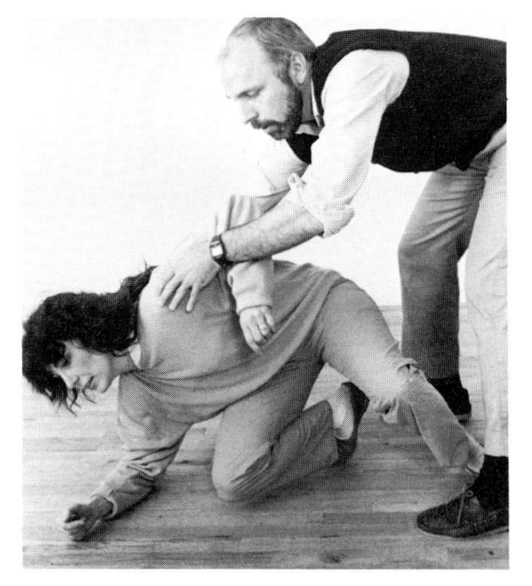

Figure 7.34 ■ Man following.

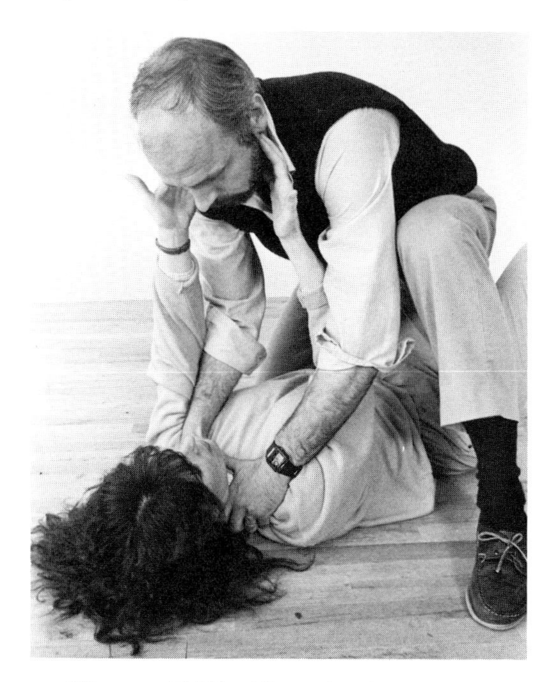

Figure 7.35 ■ Thumbs to eyes.

Rear Choke with Forearm

With this choke, the male will be directly behind you with his head over either your right or left shoulder. This choke will feel very powerful but it is no more effective than the fingers. (Fig. 7.36.)

The response to this type of choke is the same as when he uses his hands. Drop your shoulder and turn toward his hand. At best, you will only be able to get one hand in position to attack. Your response should be to reach over your shoulder and drive the thumbs into the male's eyes. (Fig. 7.37).

Because the man is always very close to this type of choke, he will be very susceptible to this attack. If, by chance, you cannot effectively reach the man's eyes, attack the testicles. (Fig. 7.38.) Once contact has been made with the testicle, turn and follow up with attack to the eyes. (Fig. 7.39.)

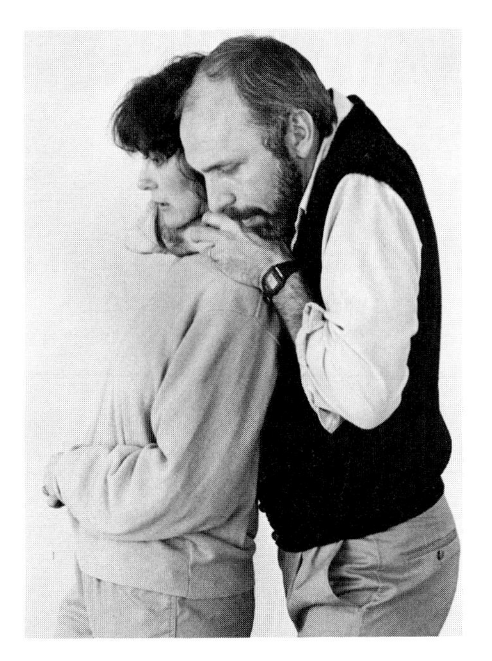

Figure 7.36 ▪ Being grabbed.

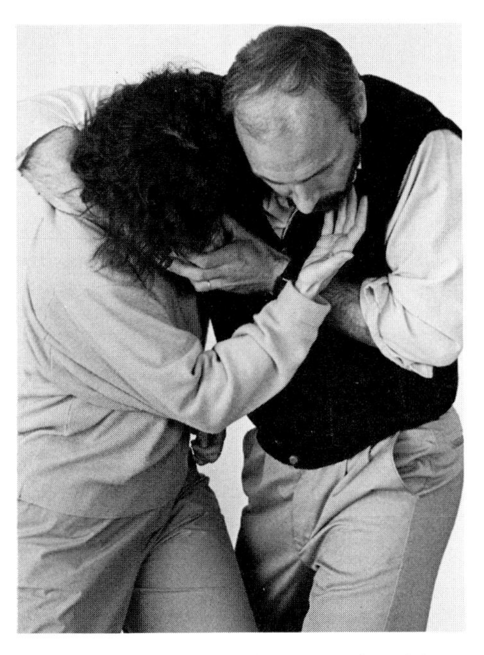

Figure 7.37 ▪ Reach over shoulder.

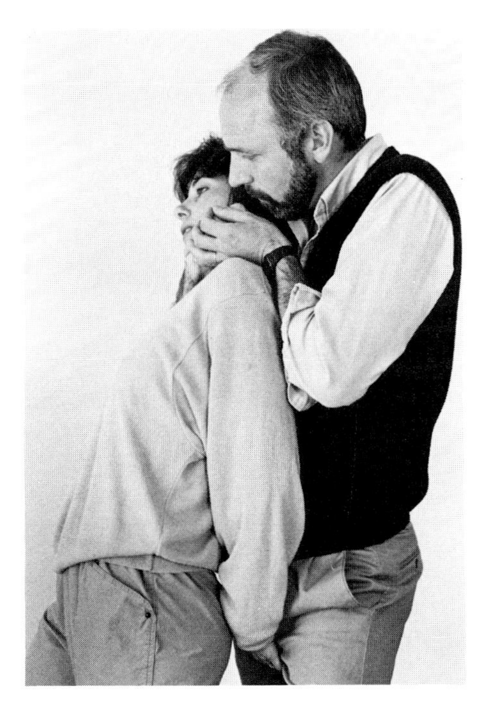

Figure 7.38 ▪ Reach for testicle.

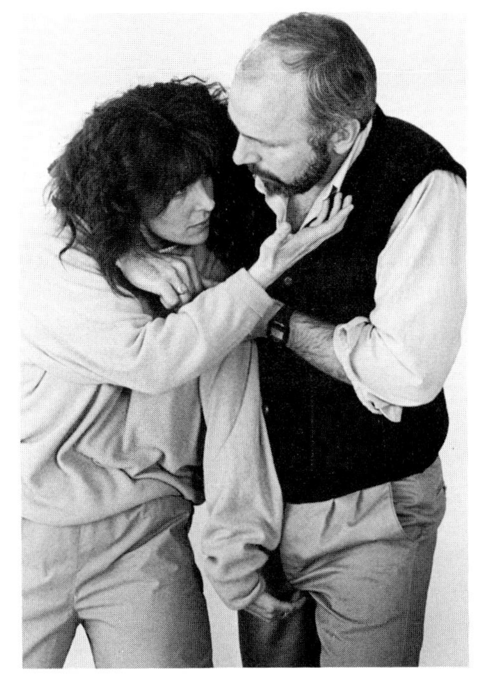

Figure 7.39 ▪ Man incapacitated—turn and follow-up to the eyes.

Garrote

The most painful and effective choke, occurs when the male uses nylons, a piece of rope, or other types of straps to choke his victim. It is much more painful because the area of pressure is so small. (Fig. 7.40.)

This is perhaps the easiest method of strangulation to get out of, if you do not panic. Your response should be, simply turn and attack the eyes. (Fig. 7.41.) You will feel no resistance to your turn because there is no friction created by the strap. Try it—you will see how simple it really is! As soon as the pressure is felt, immediately turn bringing your hands to the male's jaws. Once there, drive the thumbs into the eye sockets. *YOU WILL WIN!*

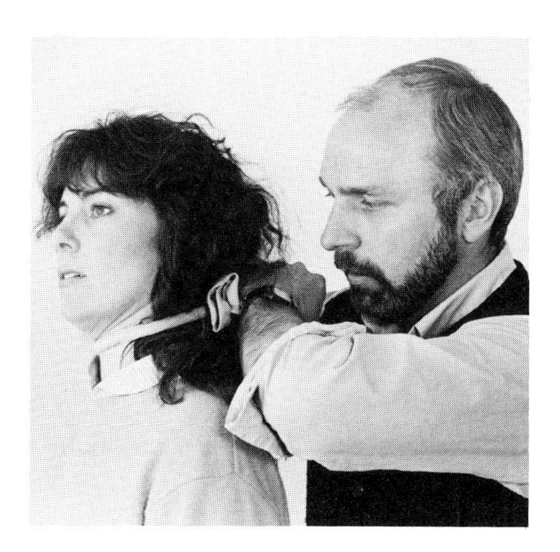

Figure 7.40 ■ Strap in place.

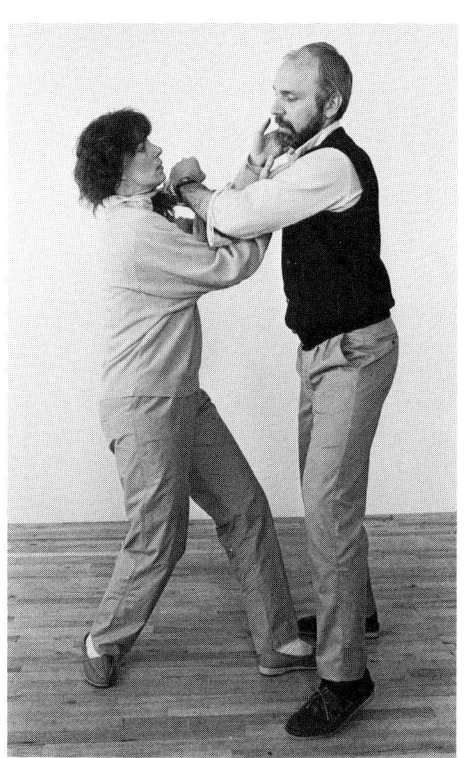

Figure 7.41 ■ Turning and attacking.

Summary of Strangulations

It is imperative that you remember that the only way to beat a choke, is to eliminate the person performing the choke. Attack the source! No matter what the situation, attack the male. You are not helpless!

Most rapists do not choke. However, if one does, it is almost always in a face-to-face position. Gain control of your body and bring your hands up to the jaw line; then drive the thumbs into the eyes.

If the choke is from the rear, attempt to turn to face the male; then attack. If you cannot turn—reach.

You must practice these responses, in order to use them in a stress situation. The more realistic your practice, the less chance of panic if in an actual situation.

GROUND SITUATIONS

Often, in attack situations, women are thrown or knocked to the ground. I have found that, generally, if able to, they often assume a face down defensive position. This is not the position most rapists would force a woman into. It is also the *worst* position for you because you have no leverage and are unable to attack. (Figs. 7.42 and 7.43.)

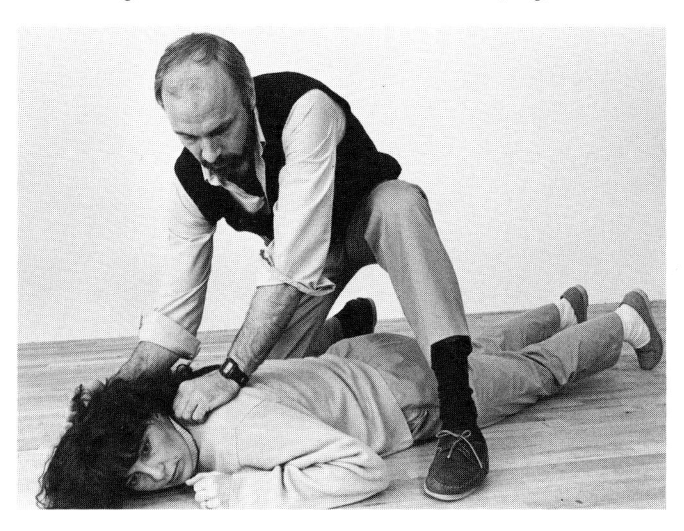

Figure 7.42 ■ Face down.

Facing the ground to avoid the assault puts you in an extremely vulnerable position. So, if thrown or knocked to the ground, the first thing you **must** do is *get to your back!*

If the male attacks you while you are on the ground, your response should be the same as when you are standing. Bring your fingertips to the male's jaw line and then drive the thumbs into the eyes. There is no chance that his attack will continue.

Many females ask how they would do this if the male was pinning down their arms. (Fig. 7.44.)

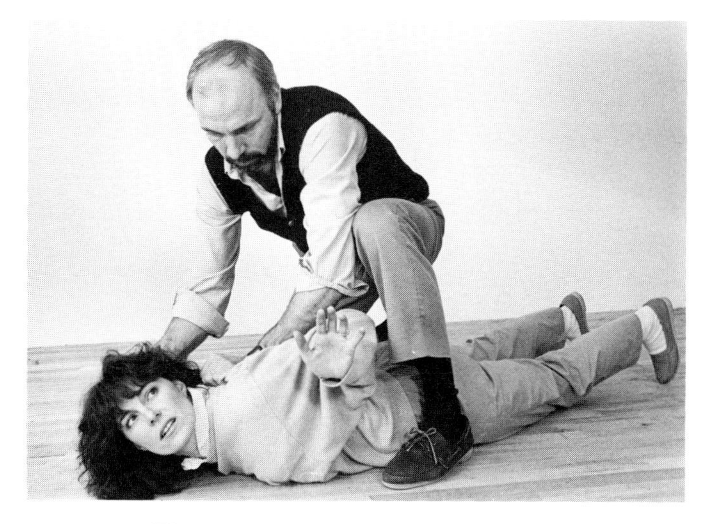

Figure 7.43 ■ Unable to reach

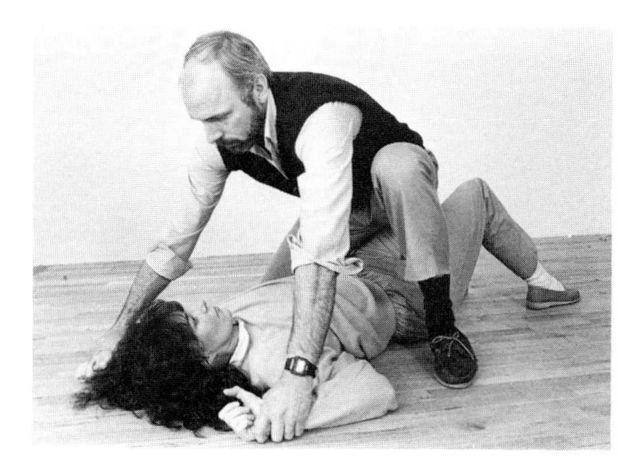

Figure 7.44 ■ Female's arms being pinned down.

Very simply, if the male is pinning your arms, it will be very difficult for him to achieve penetration. Unless you are both naked and his penis erect, there will be a time, realistically, when he will have to let go. At that time, you attack. (Figs. 7.45 and 7.46.)

Being patient is essential in many situations. If you are not being hurt, and there is a chance that you can use the psychological principles of Control, use them. At worst, this gives you some time to prepare for your counter-attack. At best, it will prevent the rape without your having to resort to the use of your body as a weapon.

Face Up

Ground situations can be broken into two types: face up and face down. As was previously stated, always try to assume a face up position.

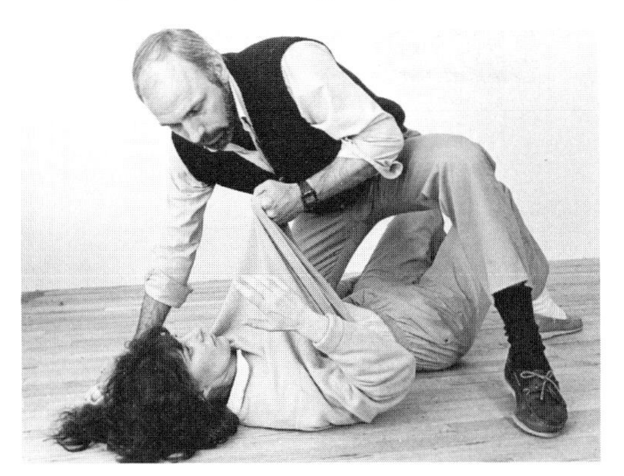

Figure 7.45 ■ Picture of pinning.

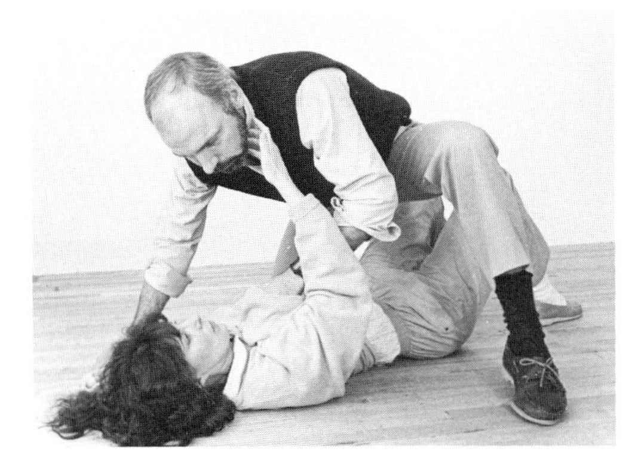

Figure 7.46 ■ Picture of male letting go to drop.

No matter how the male is attempting to strangle or strike, you will have one or both of his vital areas open for attack. (Figs. 7.47 and 7.48.) Remember, over 70 percent of all sexual assaults involve oral sex. Therefore, most of the time, the male will be exposing himself to attack.

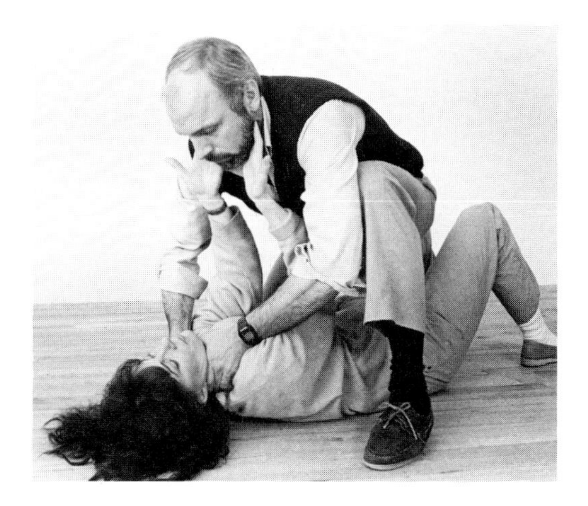

Figure 7.47 ■ Attacking eyes.

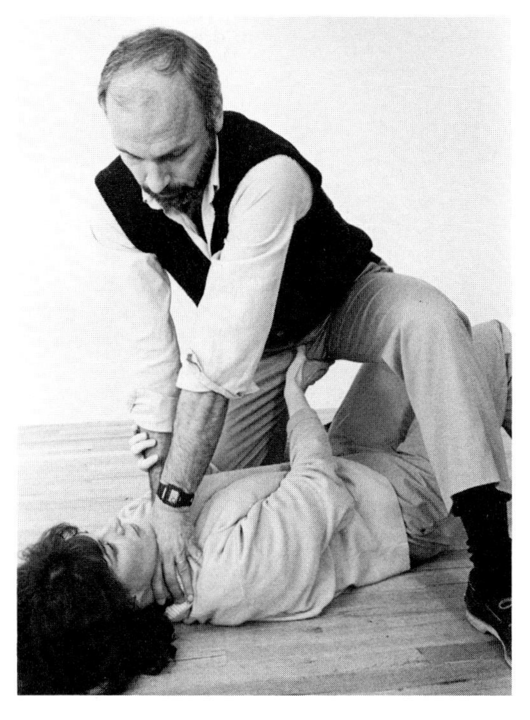

Figure 7.48 ■ Attacking testicles.

A face-up position is much like a standing, face-to-face position. The only difference is that, on the ground, you are in a stable position and the groin would be more exposed to attack. So, in any life-threatening, ground situation in which you are face-up, attack the eyes. (Fig. 7.49.)

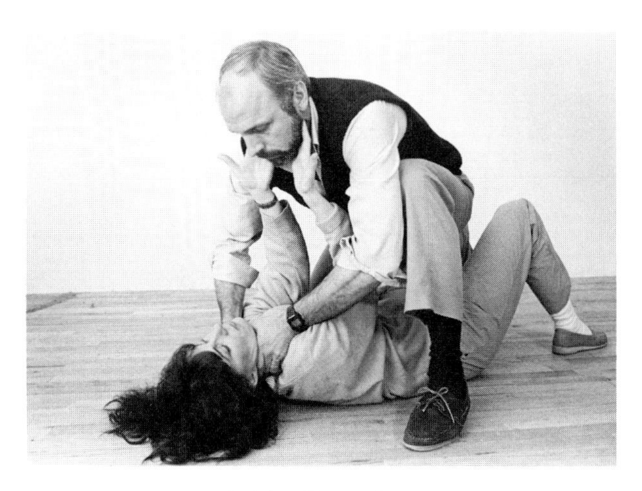

Figure 7.49 ■ Thumbs to eyes.

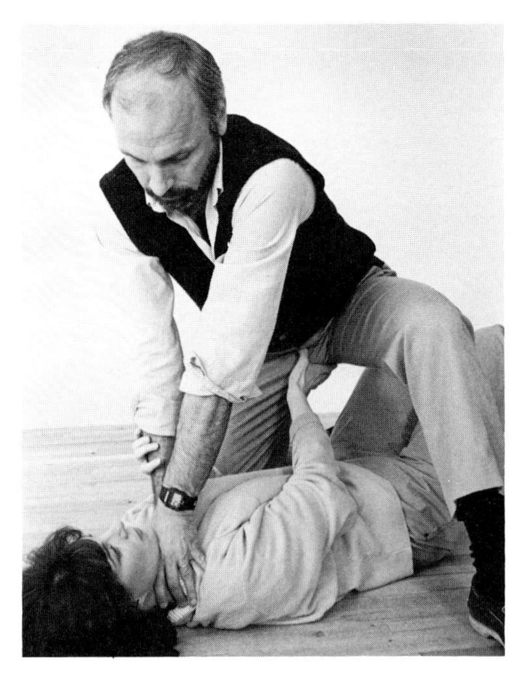

Figure 7.50 ■ Testicles.

If you cannot reach the eyes, attack the testicles (Fig. 7.50), and follow-up with attacking the eyes. (Fig. 7.51.) You always follow-up with the eyes, unless you can quickly determine and be sure that you did actually crush a testicle. When a man's genitals are exposed, this is simple. However, if he is wearing tight pants, it is difficult to get to a testicle.

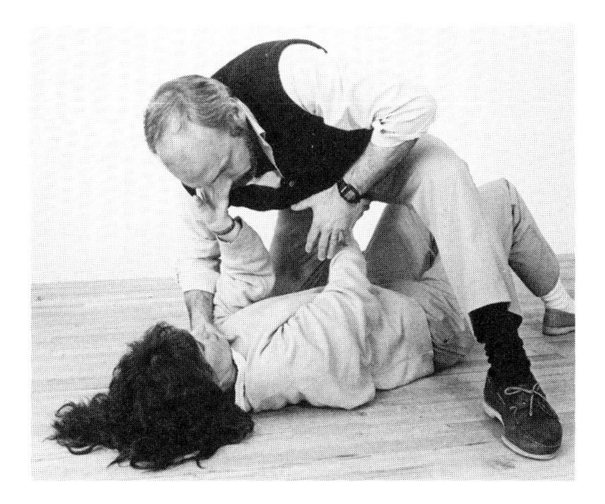

Figure 7.51 ■ Testicles follow-up to the eyes.

Face Down

Being attacked while in a face down position on the ground is very rare. Generally, as I mentioned before, it occurs because the woman rolls to the face down position. If, however, it does happen, what should you do?

This position is the most difficult one to get out of. Your goal is always to attack, but getting to an attack position is very, very difficult due to the lack of leverage you have from the face down position.

The first thing you must keep in mind, if put in this position, is that you have to move, and move quickly and continuously until you are in a position to attack one of the vital areas. Moving slowly or not

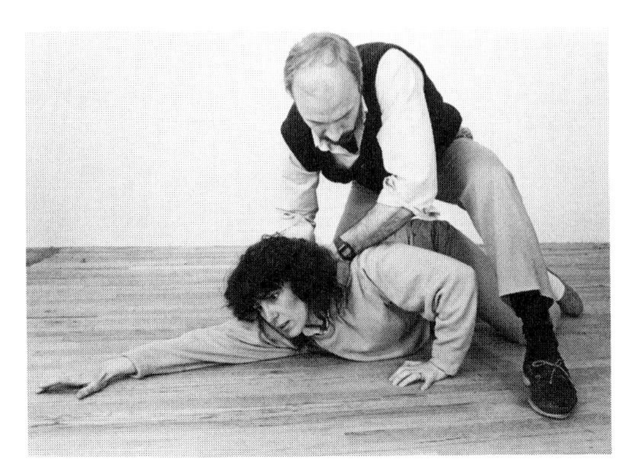

Figure 7.52 ■ Man on top—left arm moves forward.

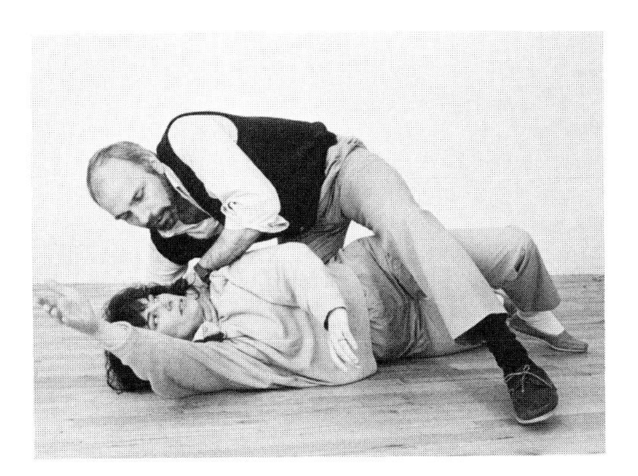

Figure 7.53 ■ Right arm bends, right leg bends—push with arm.

moving at all allows the man to tighten his grip. Whether the man is choking with his fingers or forearm, you should quickly throw one arm forward (Fig. 7.52), while bending the leg on the opposite side in order to be able to push. You should push with that forward arm. (Fig. 7.53.)

What you are attempting to do is get in a position to attack. It may mean that you are face up on top of the man (Fig. 7.54), or turned sideways and attacking. (Fig. 7.55.)

Regardless, your goal is to get to a position where you can effectively reach the eyes or groin—no more and no less!

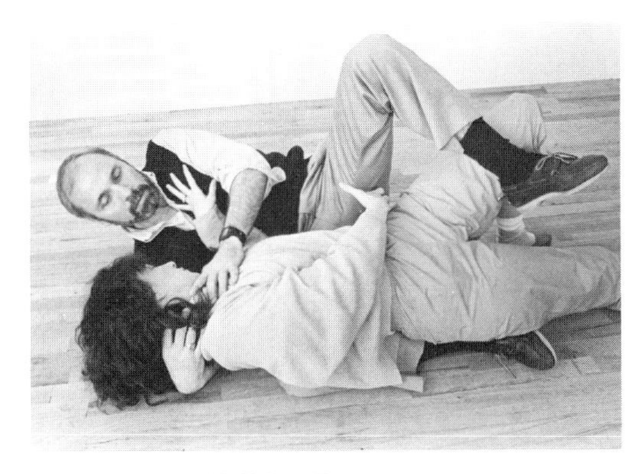

Figure 7.54 ■ Face up on top, reaching for testicle.

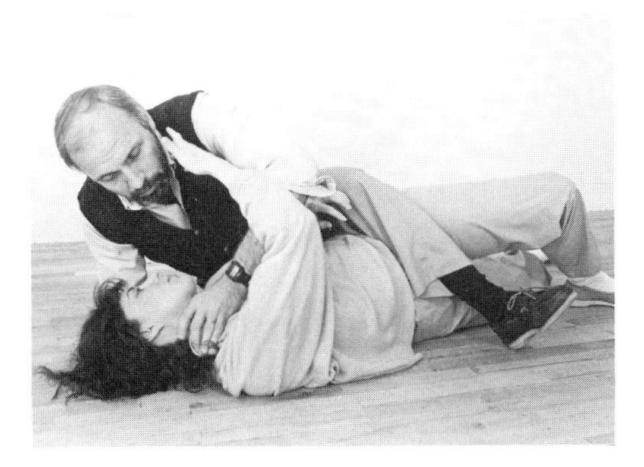

Figure 7.55 ■ Sideways attacking.

Ground Situations Summary

In any ground situation your prime purpose is to put yourself in a position from which you can use the techniques that will completely incapacitate the male. Do not attempt defense by turning over to your stomach or by trying to pry off whatever is choking you. Be aggressive—do not stop moving and fighting until you have completely incapacitated the male.

WHAT DO YOU DO IF HE HAS A WEAPON?

Often, in sexual assault situations, the male will display a weapon or threaten you with the fact that he has one (though you may not be able to see it). Whether he is a Type I or Type II, it is very possible that a weapon will be present. The difference is that a Type I uses it only as a threat, whereas, a Type II uses it as a threat and is also willing to carry out the threat and use it.

By staying relatively calm and manipulating the situation, most females can get the male to put the weapon aside. You have to convince him that it is to his advantage to put it down—be sexually explicit as to what you will do, and how much better you can perform if the threat of a weapon isn't present. Say to the male, "Please don't hurt me! I'll do whatever you say. You don't really need that knife (gun, etc.), to control me, do you?" Think about it! You are putting him in a position in which he would be degrading himself if he kept the weapon. If he keeps the weapon out, he would be admitting to himself that he is afraid of you—something no rapist could admit.

Several students of mine have been in situations in which a weapon was present. *All* were able to get the male to put the weapon down using these tactics. One such student entered her apartment after work one night and found a male waiting for her. He had a knife and told her he would use it if she did not cooperate (intimidation). It turned out that the man worked at the garage where she had her car serviced. The man, a Type II, selected her because he knew that she lived alone (vulnerable). He held the knife in front of her and demanded that she take her clothes off. Realizing that she would not be able to use Control, she decided to manipulate the man into putting the knife down. She told the man, "Please, don't kill me. I'll do what you ask, but it would be easier to respond if you put the knife down. Besides, a big man like you doesn't need a knife to control me, do you?" He put the knife down and she proceed to take her dress off. She then told the man that she would help him undress. In playing along, she was defusing aggression and setting him up to use her body as a weapon. After she got his pants and underwear off, she started to stroke his genital area. She held one of his testicle and squeezed as hard and fast as she could. The male screamed and grabbed himself.

She rushed next door to call the police. When they arrived, the man was in great pain and shock. This woman saved herself from being a victim by thinking and manipulating the male and the situation.

Remember that when dealing with a man who has a weapon, you have three objectives: the first is to be sexually explicit and make him believe it is to his advantage to put the weapon down. Second, to put him in a position in which he will humiliate himself if he continues to threaten you with the weapon (for example, "You don't really need that gun to control me, do you?"), and third, manipulate so that you can do one of the two complete incapacitators.

SUMMARY—COMPLETE INCAPACITATION

Remember, this "C" is used if Confidence, Control and Transition fail, or if the male is using life-threatening techniques against you. Complete incapacitation is your goal. This is accomplished by either driving your thumbs into the eye sockets or crushing a testicle. *Any* other techniques, such as striking at the eyes, or kicking at the groin, are relatively unsuccessful—there is too much chance for error.

It is understood that these techniques are very extreme. If you must resort to Complete Incapacitation, you can be assured that you are dealing with a violent male, who deserves the pain and damage you inflict on him in response to his attack. You never asked to be raped, and the male is responsible for his action. He does not care about your feelings or well-being in the least. This "C" has been 100 percent successful when used. No other physical techniques even come close to this success. If you have to fight, then fight to win!!

CHAPTER

8

GANG RAPE

Statistics on sexual assault clearly show that the majority of the reported assaults are committed by an individual male. When there is more than one assailant, one male generally initiates the assault, and the cohort(s) participate. In his book, *Men Who Rape,* A. Nicholas Groth wrote, "Gang rape satisfies the need of the instigator to feel in charge and in control" (page 112). This control applies to both the victim and the initiator's cohorts.

Though not particularly calming, seldom are there more than two males taking part in an assault on a female. The greater the number of males, the lower the incidence of rape. This means that there are, by far, more pair rapes than rapes involving three males or more. A fact which points out that, generally, you would be dealing with no more than two males in a potential gang rape situation.

AVOIDANCE

Devising a strategy to prevent gang rape involves the use of your first "C"—Concern. The author has found that, for the most part, gang rape occurs in three specific situations:

1. Hitchhiking. (Fig. 8.1)

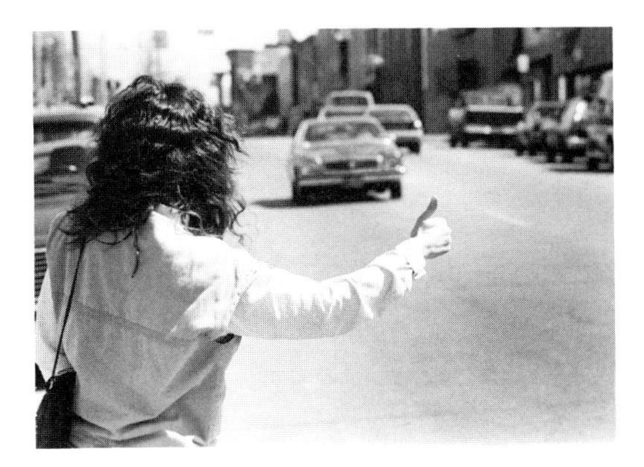

Figure 8.1 ■ Hitchhiking.

2. Attending parties where you know little about your escort and/or the other people at the party. (Fig. 8.2)

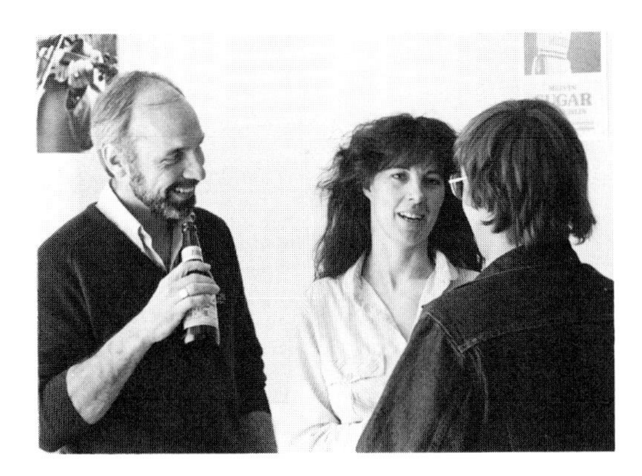

Figure 8.2 ■ Parties.

3. Being in an isolated environment that has clear potential for males congregating in groups. Places such as parks (Fig. 8.3), deserted beaches (Fig. 8.4), or vacant lots in metropolitan areas (Fig. 8.5), are examples of such environments.

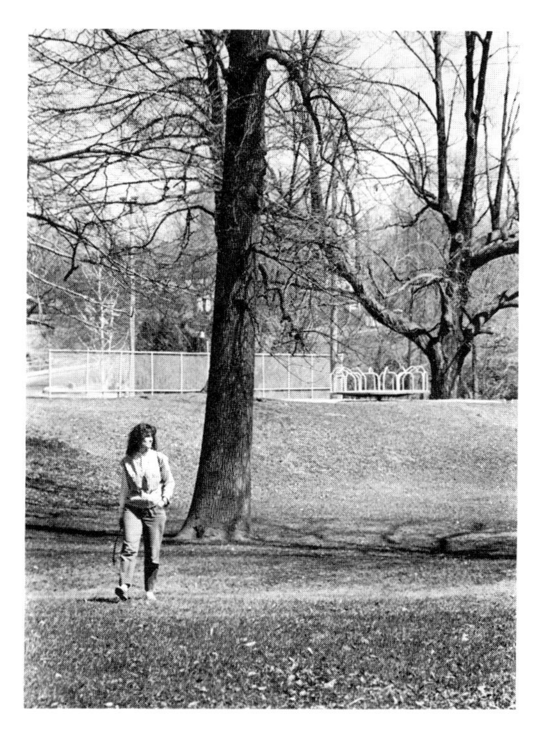

Figure 8.3 ■ Parks.

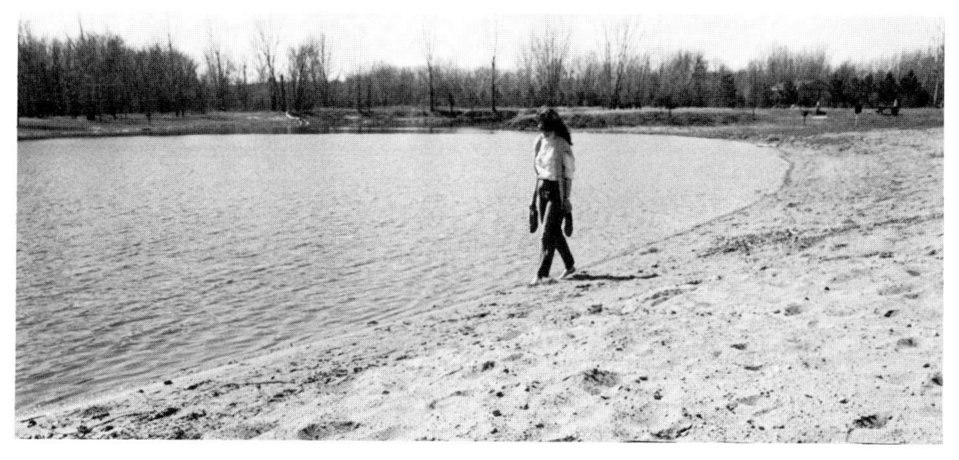

Figure 8.4 ■ Deserted beaches.

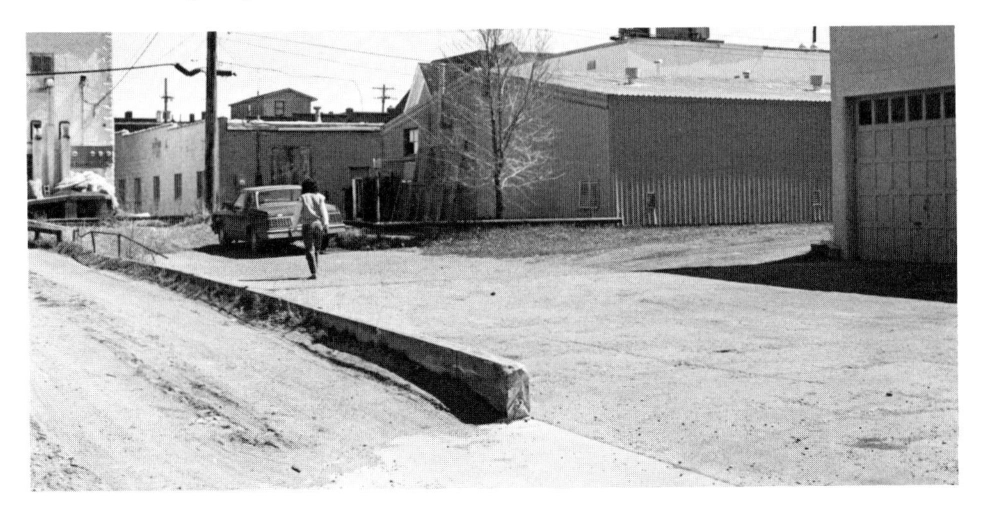

Figure 8.5 ▪ Vacant lots in metropolitan areas.

All of these environments should be easy to avoid. However, if you find yourself in a potential gang rape situation, you should attempt to defuse the aggression by remaining as calm and controlled as possible. Immediate resistance will have little, if any, effect. With this type of rape, resistance (unless completely incapacitating), will most likely provoke more violence.

Second, identify which male is the leader. He will be the one controlling the situation. Do not assume that the most boisterous male is necessarily the leader. Look for the one who directs the actions of the others.

Once you have established which one is the leader, try to get him away from the other(s). Most people have a preconceived notion that when there is more than one assailant, that they watch each other or help. Generally, this is not the case. In a majority of gang rapes, the female is alone with each male. In attempting to separate the leader from the other(s) manipulate him by saying something like, "If this is going to happen, we might as well enjoy ourselves—you don't need your friend(s) close by to feel in control, do you? It will be much better if we are by ourselves!" If this is successful, and generally, it will be, use the techniques explained in Control, to try to get away completely or around other people.

One of my former students was in a potential gang rape situation. She was targeted in a parking lot by three males in a van. She isolated the leader from the rest of the males, and convinced him to drive her to a local bar where she could get some of her female friends to take part in the "party". Once they were in the bar, she ran into the bathroom, locked the door, and screamed for the police. The bartender was not sure what was going on, but called the police anyway. She gave the police the van's license number, and shortly after, the "gang" was arrested.

If the psychological techniques do not work, one of the two techniques described in Complete Incapacitation will!! By eliminating the leader, you will most likely cause the other(s) to lose their motivation due to his/their concern for the fallen leader. Immediately, get to safety.

In the unlikely event that you cannot separate the leader from the other(s), you will have to use the techniques of Control on the other(s) as well. If you find that you cannot get away or around other people, completely incapacitate the leader or first male. This will, most likely, create enough confusion and loss of confidence for you to get away.

If the other(s) become violent, you must fight to eliminate the threat with either of the two techniques in the fourth 'C'. As long as you have hands, and males have eyes and testicles, you have the means to protect yourself.

Another former student found herself in a situation where she could not get the leader away from the other male. The psychological techniques were not working, and she realized she would have to completely incapacitate one or both of the males. She manipulated the males into a position where she had one of her hands near the face of the leader and the other hand on a testicle of the follower. She counted to three to herself and simultaneously crushed the testicle and drove her thumb into an eye. She defeated and successfully incapacitated both males.

SUMMARY

Remember, most gang assaults involve two males—a leader and a follower! They find targets in specific environmental situations. So, try to avoid these situations. If targeted, use the third 'C'—Control first and keep the use of your body as a weapon as your "trump card".

There will be a dominant male—gear yourself toward defeating him!

CHAPTER

9

REPORTING THE ATTEMPT

The successful avoidance of an assault should be followed by a report to the police. There has been, and there still is, a great deal of stereotyping in the attitudes police have toward victims of rape. At one time, the victim was looked at with a skeptical eye. Today, however, the majority of police officers in the country approach victims empathetically. True, there still exists the officer who attempts to make the woman feel responsible for what has happened, but that is not as common as it has been in the past. This is due, mainly, to the fact that officers are better educated in the dynamics of rape, and also, many of them have had relatives, friends, etc. who have been victims. They now know that women do not *ever* ask for that type of treatment.

WHY REPORT?

Why should you go to the trouble of reporting an attempted assault? This probably was not the male's first attempt at assaulting a female, and undoubtedly, it will not be his last. Whether you break out of the Rape Sequence in the Approach/Test Stage or Intimidation Stage, the information you give the police can greatly aid in the apprehension and conviction of the male. True, breaking away in the Approach/Test Stage doesn't allow you to do much more than corroborate information the police have gathered from other targeted females. However, if you break away in the Intimidation Stage, it is likely that you could press charges for verbal assault or threats against your person. Either way, you can help with an artist's sketch, corroborate information given by other victims, and help the police put together a more accurate profile. The bottom line is, that the only way to prevent rape and get the male off the street and away from other females, is to *get involved!*

WHAT INFORMATION WILL THEY WANT?

When reporting the attempt to the police, they will probably have a list of questions they would like you to answer if possible. I believe it is most helpful if you can organize your thoughts ahead of time. For example:

1. How were you targeted?

    - Location of attempt.

    - How did you happen to be at that location?

    - Were you on foot, in a car, in your home?

    - Were other people around?

2. What methods did he use to approach and talk with you.

   - Did he pose as someone like a repairperson, friend of your relations, an acquaintance, etc.?
   - What did he say?

3. If the Rape Sequence got as far as the Intimidation Stage, what happened?

   - Did he attempt to use force? How much and how?
   - Was there a weapon or threat of one?
   - What did he say?
   - Did he threaten you?

4. A description of the assailant will also be requested by the police.

   - Height and weight?
   - Race?
   - Color of hair and eyes?
   - Build (athletic, thin, fat, muscular).
   - Clothing (shoe style is very important).
   - Clean or dirty appearance?
   - Speech characteristics (accent, etc.).
   - Other distinguishing characteristics such as a large nose, beard, tattoo, smell, etc.

Other information which can be extremely helpful, are your perceptions of the assailant. For instance, did he seem to be afraid, calm, experienced, and did he appear to be familiar with the terrain?

All of this information, and probably more, will be compiled by the police in an effort to put together a clearer picture of the type of assailant, his habits, and patterns. The more information that can be gathered and compared, the greater the chance of apprehending the man.

SUMMARY

It is very important that you give a report to the police. If they do not have information about assaults or potential assaults, they cannot take any action. Their effectiveness is, to a great extent, determined by the public's willingness to get involved.

Whatever positive action you take can only help you to get the male off the street, and, for a period of time, eliminate the chance of another female being targeted by him.

CHAPTER

10

THE RAPE VICTIM

What do I say? How should I act? These are two common questions I am asked by friends and relatives of rape victims. The soundest, simplest advice I can give is to support the victim by never asking a "why" question.

Why did you go out by yourself? Why didn't you fight more? Why didn't you call me sooner? Why . . . why . . . why? The last thing a victim needs is for someone to question her actions. There is absolutely nothing she can do now to change what has happened. We must give support and comfort, but how?

Victims have expressed to me that they feel so out of control and afraid during the assault. Once the assault is over and they reach out to someone significant for help, that person due to anger, confusion, frustration, or fear, often reacts in ways that take from the victim rather than give support to her.

SIGNIFICANT OTHERS

I have broken the significant others into three categories. Within each category I will describe what I see as typical responses and then give recommendations.

Friends

Some do a very fine job of being empathetic and supportive, however, many do not. When a trauma such as rape occurs it is very common for female friends to ask "why" questions. The reason for this is that friends tend to set the victim up as being different from them. By asking why, for example, the victim walked back home from a party alone, the friend is really telling herself that she is different because she would know better than to do so. Establishing that the victim acted differently than you would act sets her apart from you and thus, you deny the possibility that you could be a victim.

Do not ask "why" questions and do not judge her. Rather, attempt to listen and allow her to be emotional. She is probably blaming herself and, more than anything else, needs you to sympathize and show her that she is not at fault. You should try to get her to a hospital so that her physical trauma can be treated. I advise that your next step is to call in a professional who is trained to help victims of rape.

After a few days you should still show support by asking how she is doing, etc., but you should also not allow it to consume you. Life must go on. Try to engage her in the activities you used to do prior to the assault. Victims are very sensitive to people treating them differently. I can not emphasize enough that she should see a professional to help her deal with the rape trauma common to victims.

Spouse/Boyfriend

This gets tricky because now a macho, possessive attitude comes into play. Initially, the male may be supportive in that he shows genuine concern for her. However, it is extremely common for the male to become very angry and want to "kill" the guy. Instead of receiving support, the victim, generally, feels she has to soothe the male's ego and prevent him from doing something that he may have to pay for later.

After the victim has been called upon to cool the male off, she then is often told by the male that she must press charges. I have dealt with many males who have involved the police without first asking the victim. It's control! As a male, I have been socialized to be the protector, the one to make decisions. Now, I find that I have no control. My wife/girlfriend was raped and there was nothing I could do. So, what's the next best thing? Revenge through prosecution! I am doing something! Forget about her. I need control—to feel like I'm retaliating. This is all too familiar a scenario.

Typically, within a few days, he will want to re-establish sexual relations with the victim. While she probably needs to feel secure and wanted, he needs to be reassured through sex. Quite often the two are not compatible. I wish I could say that most relationships make it through the various stages of rape trauma, but they do not. I strongly suggest that significant males be supportive and *do not* attempt to control the victim. He should bring in professional help as quickly as possible for the victim and for himself so that they may both have assistance in dealing with the trauma.

Parents

It doesn't matter what age out children are, as parents, we are concerned for their well-being. When something traumatic happens to them, we also experience trauma.

Typically, what happens if the parents are not meeting their daughter's needs first, is that the mother will listen and become emotional, calling upon the victim to comfort the mother and assure her that she, the daughter, is okay. The father, on the other hand, quite often reacts the same way as a boyfriend or husband—anger followed by the need to take action. Instead of giving support to their daughter, they take from her.

It is very common, after the initial response, for the parents to place blame on their daughter and enter into a stage where the topic is not mentioned. Often families do not want to bring in professional help because others would then know. So, the victim is expected to forget it

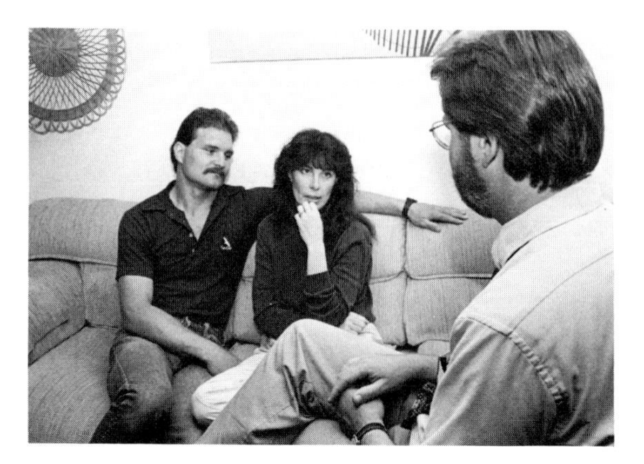

Figure 10.1 ■ Male and female with counselor.

and carry on with life. She can't talk about it so she builds walls around her emotions.

As with friends, and significant males, parents must allow the victim to talk. They must support her by listening and not judging. Finally, they should attempt to bring in a professional who can help all of them deal with the trauma.

SUMMARY

Many fine books and articles deal with the subject of rape trauma. Simply put, the victim's needs come first. No matter who she reaches out to or comes in contact with, her well being is paramount. Do not judge her, never ask "why", listen, and finally, try to bring in professional help for her, and possibly for yourself. Few of us are equipped to give anything but temporary support.

CHAPTER

11

A FINAL WORD

To effectively deal with an attempted sexual assault, first takes an acknowledgement on your part that you could be victimized. Once this is established, knowledge concerning the avoidance of rape takes on a much more important perspective. What works, what doesn't work, and why?

I have attempted to answer these questions. You have learned that there are two types of rapists. Each is motivated differently, yet all follow a pattern of behavior called the Rape Sequence. I have shown you various rape avoidance strategies and discussed why they have successes and, more importantly, why they fail.

Failure is not a word associated with the Four 'C's'. It is designed to counter the rape sequence no matter what type of rapist.

Remember 'C' #1—Concern, asks that you look at your particular lifestyle and attempt to reduce the times when you are targetable. If you find that, for whatever reason, you are exposed to a rape situation, implement the second and third 'C's'—Confidence and Control. Rapists expect you to be frightened or to fight them. By controlling the situation through these principles, you throw him off balance psychologically and are generally able to manipulate him long enough so that you can get around people. If this is not working, you move into a phase of the system called *Transition.* This is a last ditch effort to get away without having to physically harm the man. The success rates of *Control* and *Transition* increase in proportion to how well you know him.

The final course of action available to you is your fourth 'C'—*Complete Incapacitation.* You use this if *Control* and *Transition* fail or if the man does not give you a chance to use them. This option will not fail. However, it must be understood that there is a moral responsibility that goes with it. You do not play with this option!

The success of the Four 'C's' is directly related to your ability to implement them. If you give little thought to the possibility of being victimized, and if you do not engage in ongoing practice, the likelihood of successfully using the Four 'C's' is low. There are no easy answers—no guarantees. Success depends upon you!

That's it, you have it all! Mentally and physically practice your options. By rehearsing situations in your mind, the time lapse between shock, fear, and purposeful action can be shortened. You will be confident in your ability to defend yourself. You now have the option to win!

Suggested Readings

James Selkin, ''Behavioral Analysis of Rape'', unpublished research report, Violence Research Unit, Denver General Hospital, Denver, Colorado.

A. Nicholas Groth and H. Jean Birnbaum, *Men Who Rape,* New York, New York, Plenum Publishing Corporation, 1979.

R. R. Hazelwood and A. W. Burgess, Eds., *Practical Aspects of Rape Investigation: A Multidisciplinary Approach,* New York, New York, Elsevier Science Publishing Co., 1986.

Thomas Stuntz and Conrad V. Hassel, ''The Sociopath—A Criminal Enigma'', Journal of Police Science and Administration, June, 1978.

L. L. Holstrom and A. W. Burgess, ''Sexual Behavior of Assailants During Rape'', Archives of Sexual Behavior, Vol. 9, No. 5, 1980.

J. C. Coleman, et. al., *Abnormal Psychology and Modern Life,* Sixth Edition, Glenview, Illinois, Scott, Foresman, and Company, 1980.

L. L. Holstrom and A. W. Burgess, ''Rapists Talk: Linguistic Strategies to Control the Victim'', Deviant Behavior, Vol. 1, 1979.

Konrad Lorenz, *On Aggression,* New York, New York, Harcourt-Brace-Jovanovich, Inc., 1971.

Julius Fast, *Body Language,* New York, New York, Simon and Schuster, 1970.

Ann Burgess and L. L. Holstrom, ''Rape Trauma Syndrome'', American Journal of Psychiatry, No. 9, September, 1974.

R. R. Hazelwood and Joseph Harpold, ''Rape: The Dangers of Providing Confrontational Advice'', F.B.I. Law Enforcement Bulletin, June, 1986.

Menachem Amir, *Patterns in Forcible Rape,* Chicago Illinois, University of Chicago Press, 1971.

A. Nicholas Groth, Ann Wolbert Burgess, and Lynda Lytle Holstrom, ''Rape: Power, Anger, and Sexuality'', American Journal of Psychiatry, No. 11, November, 1977.